Also by Mark Lauren and Joshua Clark

You Are Your Own Gym

BODY BY YOU

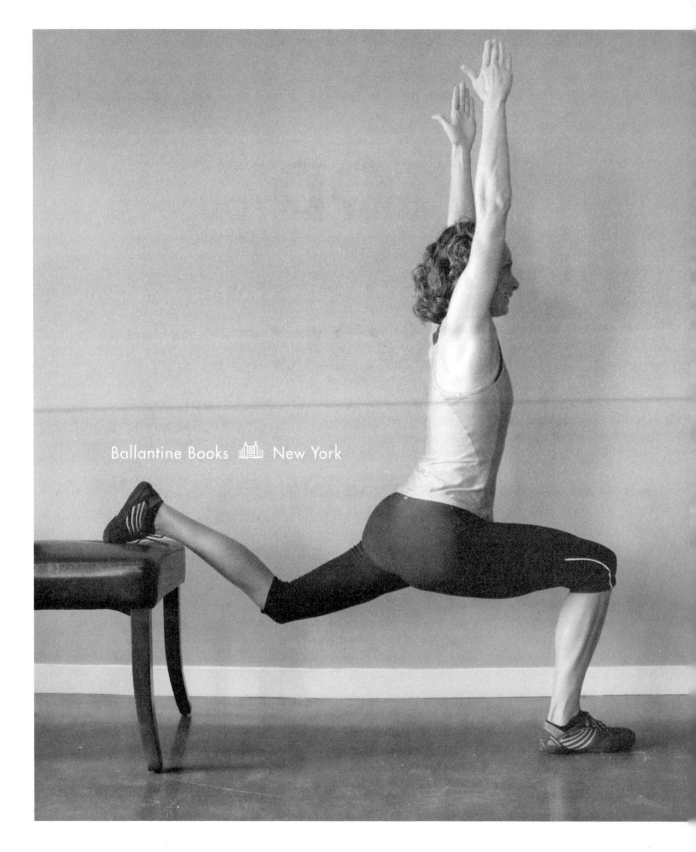

Ballantine Books 🏛 New York

BODY BY YOU

The *You Are Your Own Gym* Guide to Total Fitness for Women

Mark Lauren

with Joshua Clark

Body by You proposes a program of exercise recommendations for
the reader to follow. However, you should consult a qualified medical
professional (and, if you are pregnant, your ob-gyn) before starting this
or any other fitness program. As with any diet or exercise program,
if at any time you experience any discomfort, stop immediately
and consult your physician.

A Ballantine Books Trade Paperback Original

Published in the United States by Ballantine Books,
an imprint of The Random House Publishing Group,
a division of Random House, Inc., New York.

BALLANTINE and colophon are registered trademarks of Random House, Inc.

BODY BY YOU is a trademark of Mark Kling.

LIBRARY OF CONGRESS-CATALOGING-IN-PUBLICATION DATA
Lauren, Mark.
Body by you : the you are your own gym guide to total fitness for women /
Mark Lauren with Joshua Clark.
p.   cm.
ISBN 978-0-345-52897-1
eBook ISBN 978-0-345-52898-8
1. Physical fitness for women. 2. Exercise for women.
I. Clark, Joshua. II. Title.
GV482.L38 2013
613.7082—dc23   2012033491

Printed in the United States of America

www.ballantinebooks.com

9 8 7 6 5 4 3 2 1

Book design by Mary A. Wirth

For the countless women who helped inspire this book,
both friends and role models, and most of all for our mothers—
who are the greatest of both.

And also for the wives of military personnel. It is not the individual soldier
who makes the ultimate sacrifice in times of war. It is the families who do.
They must endure the separation of long deployments while fearing for their
beloveds' lives. And should the worst become a reality, the surviving partners
must carry on and continue to provide. For them, the struggle has just begun.

Five Things to Love About This Program

Saves money. No dues, trainers, babysitters, or home fitness equipment.

Saves time. Driving to and changing at a gym, doing cardio and weights . . . At the end of the week, you're looking at a loss of 8 to12 hours. Now, just 3 days a week, you start and about 30 minutes later you're finished. This is less than one percent of your time.

Do it anywhere. Your bedroom, hotel room, a park, roof, garage, yard, your office between meetings.

No gymbarrassment. No television shouting at you. No one watching you. No sweaty machines. No tracksuits.

Burns more fat. These exercises will crank your body's metabolism far above using weights or aerobics.

Contents

Introduction   xiii

Part I: All Body, No Bulk

1. What's Keeping You from Having the Body You Want?   3
2. Why Bodyweight Training Is the Key to Your Best Body Ever   13
3. Staying Motivated   17

Part II: The *Body by You* Program

4. Your Training Schedule   29
5. Getting Started   35
6. The Movement Categories, Progressions, and Exercises   47

Part III: *Body by You* Nutrition

7. The Basics   111
8. Read Your Food, Plan Your Food   121
9. The Top Ten Ways to Gain as Much Fat as Possible!   133

The Final Step: Independence   137
Acknowledgments   139

Introduction

For a decade I've used my bodyweight movements to create the leanest, strongest, most confident people on earth in as little time as possible. I honed the exercises in this book while preparing nearly a thousand trainees for the extreme demands of the most elite levels of the United States Special Operations community. Now the military's most advanced forces—from SEALs to Green Berets—use these movements.

This is not "boot camp" run by some gym instructor in spandex who's never laced up a pair of combat boots. This is the world's most effective and efficient workout program from someone whose day job is to physically train troops who've worn their boots through countless miles of mud, sand, and snow. Cool high-tech gear and weapons aside, the things that most determine a soldier's survival and victory are physical fitness and resolve: my areas of expertise.

My first book, *You Are Your Own Gym*, owes its continued success among popular fitness books to teaching people to exercise alone, anywhere, anytime. I've heard from countless readers who tell me that they have followed my program and now look and feel the best they ever have in their lives. While this feedback is extremely uplifting, gratifying, and personally inspiring, it's also not much of a surprise, considering I've already seen the effects on the hundreds of troops I've trained.

You Are Your Own Gym remains the "bible of bodyweight exercises."

Through its 125 exercises, comprehensive training tools, and workout routines, it has helped sculpt the physiques of tens of thousands of people. While many women have told me of their great success with *You Are Your Own Gym*, I've also heard that it didn't always meet a woman's needs and concerns—from having less time to work out to wanting to address different physical goals. I tailored *Body by You* to those needs. Some of the movements I share in this book are new, and some are updated or adapted from exercises in *You Are Your Own Gym*. Taken as a whole, these exercises will guide you from where you are now to where you want to be, to look and feel the best you ever have in your life. You'll find that the workout never stays the same for long and the results—toned arms, flatter abs, tighter buns, leaner legs, and curves in all the right places—just keep on coming. I'm not going to show you how to "lose" the fat on your belly or thighs. I'm going to show you how to—as we say in the military—"engage it for permanent termination."

Let's state the obvious: Women and men are different in lots of different ways. But the reality is that women's muscles are made up of the same fibers as men's. Our fat cells are identical. Our hormonal differences are what raise an interesting issue. Male testosterone levels make large muscles possible. Without the same high levels, women can't bulk up in the same way as men—so stop worrying about that. What you *will* get out of my method is a solid foundation of strength, the kind of strength that leads to a lean physique and powerful athleticism. You will find the natural athlete that lies at your core. Feel the pride and joy in challenging yourself to rise beyond your own expectations and the peace and strength and beauty that come from it.

Physical ability represents not only your mastery of the world around you but also of yourself. An essential source of self-confidence is pride and control over a finely tuned body. Follow my program and you won't ever have to run to anyone else for help because you're not strong enough or don't have the endurance. You'll be fit enough not only to cope with anything you want but to enjoy anything you want. You won't have to think if you *can* do something, only if you *want* to do something.

I like to say that *you* are the only piece of exercise "equipment" you will ever need to be in the best shape of your life. You now hold in your hands the only user's manual for that equipment you will ever need. Face it: For thousands of years, humanity's greatest female physical specimens—from ancient Greece's female athletes to tomorrow's G.I. Janes—have *not* relied on Gold's Gyms or weights in their basements. Male or female, the human body doesn't require machines and dumbbells (or cardio!) in order to stay fit. Free yourself from the dependency on gadgets, trainers, and common misconceptions. They are *all* crutches, keeping you from getting into the best shape possible.

This book will not teach you to move through the gym with ease. It will teach you to move through life with ease. You will learn to use the body you have to build the body you want. With just a small commitment of time—without having to go to and from a gym—you can fit this program into even your busiest schedule. The effort and time you put into my program will not be great, but the benefits you get out of it will be.

This book is about you. You are the boss now. Your destiny is controlled by you. Not by your gym. Not by complicated fitness equipment. Not by dumbbells. Not by benches and bouncy balls and treadmills and yoga mats and infomercial contraptions. Not by some trainer. Not by your friends. Just by you.

It's about you being leaner, stronger, more confident and energetic. You having the best body you can. You getting these results faster than ever before. And sustaining them as long as you live.

I offer you all body: a flatter stomach, tighter thighs and glutes, more-toned arms, sculpted shoulders, stronger pecs to give your bosom a boost, a back that turns heads when you wear an evening dress, legs that look great in a pair of shorts. Everyone around you, both men and other women, will notice the changes in your body. You will look as strong on the outside as you feel on the inside.

I offer you no bulk: No filler. No flab. No gab. No bloated chapters with unnecessary chatter. I offer you only what you'll need to look and feel as good as possible. I want to free up the rest of your time to do more of whatever you enjoy.

Looking good is not some mysterious, complicated, grueling process. Being truly in shape is not a fantasy destination. Even becoming an elite athlete, if that's what you want to do, is surprisingly simple. All you need are a few minutes of strength training a day and a good understanding of the basics of nutrition. You find those minutes, and I'll show you what to do. You give me just a little more time, and I'll explain the nutrition basics that will simplify your eating choices for good.

As much as I want you to look and feel good, this book is also ultimately about saving your life. It's a plain fact that unfit people are at far greater risk of suffering painful illnesses, immobility, and disease, from osteoporosis and arthritis to mortal threats like heart attack. Physical inactivity is the cause of one third of all deaths due to diabetes, colon cancer, and heart disease. We are all training for our lives. Whether you like it or not, life is the ultimate sport; you must approach it as an athlete would.

Even if you haven't lifted anything but groceries in years, this book is the first to offer you total fitness independence. It will shatter old stereotypes and open your eyes to previously unimaginable possibilities of female athleticism. You will be training your body to do what it couldn't before. To use muscles it didn't before. To be fit and therefore look better than ever before.

It sounds hokey, but I truly believe everyone possesses not only an inner beauty but an outer one as well. There are not ugly and pretty people. There are only *fit* people and *unfit* people. No one who is fit is not beautiful in her own way.

Whether leading training sessions or missions, competing in Thai boxing competitions, or enjoying the few vacations I get, I've been fortunate to travel a good part of this earth. From visiting my relatives in the Philippines and Germany—where I lived until I was nine, without speaking a word of English—to my military tours throughout the Middle East and Asia, I've met people in just about every shape and form in which they exist. And never, not ever, have I found a kind of people that is not breathtakingly gorgeous. Of course, all the world's nationalities and ethnicities meet and mix in America, more than in any other country, and the results all are beautiful.

What's *not* beautiful to me is the typical advertising of women. I see it in all the world's cities now: enormous billboards cast two stories high, parading some phony Western ideal of beauty—tall, bone thin, and mainly white. And it's sad and a bit maddening to see so many millions of innately beautiful women walking the streets below, trying to emulate this ridiculous, marketing-driven ideal.

Most models have a body type possessed by a minority, mostly by very young and naturally thin women, and only for a genetically select few is it carried into their thirties, forties, fifties, sixties, and beyond without proper exercise and nutrition. From an early age, women are conditioned to value this standard, which is extremely difficult (if not impossible) to achieve and maintain.

And it's not only an unachievable standard but an incredibly unhealthy one too. These models are generally devoid of any athleticism. Instead, they're simply thin. And so women try to achieve this body type through weight loss alone. This is a large contributing factor to the ineffective, unhealthy fitness methods used by many women today, mainly dieting and aerobic activity. But while some media images continue to promote unhealthy, unnatural standards of feminine beauty, the days of the waif model are numbered. We're seeing more-athletic women in advertising and even in fashion magazines now. For the first time, our culture is embracing strong women in the way that we have men for so long. We are finally embracing real beauty.

No matter your height or heritage, bone structure or age, an athletic body shows to all how beautiful you are. And this strong outer self will lead you to a powerful inner one.

Everyone has her own beauty. So reveal yours. Be strong. Be beautiful. Be yourself. Shine.

Certain exercises feature a QR (quick response) code on the page. Using any barcode scanner app on your smartphone or tablet, scan the app and you'll be directed to an exercise demo video so you can follow along! If you don't have a barcode scanner on your device, visit the YouTube channel here: http://bit.ly/ReJalT

More than revolution, this book is evolution. Since the dawn of civilization, we have slowly grown weaker as our shelters have grown stronger. Physically, we've not just stepped down on the evolutionary ladder, we've fallen off and landed in La-Z-Boys, office chairs, and workout benches. This book will not only get you back on that ladder, it'll help you take the next step up.

We need to regain our leaner, stronger, primal bodies. It's a great irony: The only way for us to physically evolve is to *reject* technology, such as the computerized *Tron*-like toys that clutter fitness centers and make women look like cyborgs. But what we should not reject is the millennia's worth of knowledge, experience, and expertise we have gained in sports science, which culminates here, rendered into the quick, comprehensive, and comprehensible program you now have in your hands.

Get ready to evolve.

PART I

All Body, No Bulk

What's Keeping You from Having the Body You Want?

From talking to women all over the country about their fitness goals and their workout practices, it seems to me that one of the greatest obstacles to having a lean, strong body is a woman's reluctance to focus on her own needs. Between families and/or careers, many women are busier now than ever before. They are so focused on others that they have little time for themselves.

Here's what I find ironic: Giving so much of yourself to those around you may in fact be making life more difficult, not easier, for them. Certainly that's the case when it comes to your long-term health. Put it this way: Do you really want your loved ones to someday visit you in the hospital rather than your home? Do you want your grandchildren to know you only in a wheelchair? Your focus on others at the expense of your own health perpetuates an endlessly repeating, zero-sum game; no one wins. You spend time and energy taking care of others, who later must spend their time and energy taking care of you. You have limited your life's potential so that they may have a good life, but when the time comes, they, too, have to limit their potential, not only caring for the next generation but caring for you.

While there is no actual fountain of youth, exercise has proven over and over again to be the closest thing. Becoming a stronger, leaner you *now* paves the way for a brighter, stronger future for all those around you. If you care about their happiness, *care about your own.*

HOOYA!

Having children must shift from being an excuse not to exercise to being the primary reason to exercise—a reason to look, feel, and perform at your best. You owe it to those around you as much as you owe it to yourself. Exercise to make your life, and that of your children, easier. Lead by example.

But let's say you *do* make time for yourself and you *do* go to an exercise class or circuit-train on gym equipment regularly. Is that really working for you? Are you in the best shape of your life? Do you feel athletic and in control? I didn't think so.

In 2012, Americans spent over $20 billion in health-club memberships. But I say that savvy marketing is robbing you of cash and buying you very little. Twice as many people belong to gyms as they did twenty years ago. And yet obesity is skyrocketing. This sends a clear message: What we're doing is *not* working.

I take issue with the kinds of exercise you'll get at the gym (more on that below), but in my view gyms are also guilty of exploiting the belief that women like exercising in group classes because they are social creatures at heart. They trick you into replacing real social time with climbing into spandex and futilely sweating with others to techno music while an instructor soothes you with superficial support.

Okay, group activities can be fun. But there are far more fun ways to hang with your friends or meet new people than getting stinky in a fitness center, don't you think? Furthermore, why would you want to mold your day's valuable free time around someone else's schedule when you could work out when it's convenient *for you*? Why listen to their music when you can choose your own? Why pay for encouragement when you can have real results? Break away from the comfort of being in a group, and find comfort in your own body.

The Myth of Cardio Efficiency

So why do some people still sweat it out to techno tunes in crowded aerobics classes or cycle to nowhere on stationary bikes? Answer: the calorie defense. That is, they think that aerobic activity burns a ton of calories. But here's the unfortunate truth: If you put whole milk and sugar in your morning latte, *boom*, you've just consumed more calories than you burned during an average cardio workout. Cardio is simply an incredibly ineffective use of your time—an average of only 200 calories burned per 45 minutes of activity.

Cardio exercise keeps you weak and pudgy because it *doesn't build muscle*. In fact, cardio exercise can cause a *loss* of muscle, because your body will shed anything it's not using. And if you're only doing cardio, you're

HOOYA!

It's time to take out the garbage. Toss out what you've been taught about "women's fitness." Throw out the baby weights. Step away from the treadmill. Get off the wheel-less bike. Quit hopping around in some class. Don't be seduced by empty glam-magazine promises and the useless fitness gadgets on the market. Don't waste your *time* and *money* on fitness-center memberships. Remember, the most advanced fitness machine is the one thing you are never without: your own body.

not using most of your muscle mass. If your goal is to get lean, you need to build muscle, plain and simple.

Here's what I want to make clear: Your focus should not be on the few calories you burn *during* exercise; instead, I want you to focus on the metabolic boost that muscles give you the rest of the time, even while you sleep. Gaining muscle through strength training is the key to losing weight.

Think of your muscular system as a motor that requires fuel (calories) while both working and idling. On average, each pound of muscle burns ten calories a day at complete rest. That's 3,650 calories a year—more than a pound of fat, which clocks in at 3,500 calories. Adding just a few pounds of muscle is equivalent to upgrading to a stronger motor that burns more fuel.

Not only is aerobic activity ineffective at improving body composition or overall fitness, it's also not nearly as safe as most people believe it to be. Its highly repetitive nature makes the risk of overuse injuries high. The thousands or even millions of identical repetitions that you undertake over the years are likely to cause unnoticed cumulative stress on joints, until chronic injuries eventually surface.

Sure, there are the few genetically exceptional people who can run, cycle, or hop around for a decade without problems, but these people are a small minority. For every success story of someone who spent a lifetime pounding the pavement or hunching over a bike, there are many more for whom injuries resulted—too often, ironically—in a loss of mobility.

I cringe every time I see an overweight man or woman running to get in shape, bouncing up and down, with knees and elbows all going their own way. Without first developing a foundation of strength and stability, running or jumping around in an aerobics class is a formula for failure.

HOOYA!

The body adapts to whatever stress we place on it, and initially difficult and energy-consuming tasks quickly become less difficult as we learn efficient motor patterns. Unless you increase intensity continually, the calorie expenditure of an activity will decrease as your movement proficiency increases. This is why aerobics instructors are often not as lean as you would expect. They have become so efficient at that particular type of activity that they are no longer burning very many extra calories doing it. This is also why trotting along at the same pace day in, day out, on machines such as treadmills takes you nowhere, literally and figuratively.

The Myth of the "Fat-Burning Zone"

But what about the magic "fat-burning zone"? If you've used a stationary bike or elliptical machine, you've seen the "target heart rate" monitors that encourage you to exercise in the fat-burning zone. The marketing logic on this is that when you get your heart rate between 120 and 140 beats per minute through light, prolonged activity, you are oxidizing fat to fuel your movement instead of using sugars and phosphates, which is what more-intense activity involves.

Unfortunately, while a fat-burning zone sounds like where you want to be, this is one of the biggest hoaxes going, and as long as you subscribe to it—and keep plugging away at 120 to 140 beats per minute—you'll be going nowhere fast.

While it's true that high-intensity activity doesn't burn much fat *during* the very short interval of the actual workout, the thing left unsaid is that it burns fat for many hours *after* the workout in order to replenish the sugars and phosphates, rebuild muscle, strengthen joints, and increase bone density. Low-intensity activity, on the other hand, causes none of this "after burn," and calorie usage returns to normal almost immediately after you step off the machine you're on. The fat you mobilized during the low-intensity, fat-burning-zone workout is almost negligible.

Honestly, if you want to lose weight by running, for example, you need to run hard, and I can tell you from many miles of personal experience that there are few things more grueling than prolonged intense aerobic activity. Just ask some of my Combat Control trainees. You can lose some pounds, but it's a terribly inefficient way of doing it, and you have to stay far above the fat-burning zone.

Activity in the "zone" is best reserved for warm-ups, cooldowns, active recovery between days of strength training, and the development of movement proficiency for specific endurance sports.

The Myth of Nautilus

You are not a cyborg! You don't need machines to move your muscles through a fixed range of motion. Besides improving strength, endurance, and body composition, your training should develop stability, effective movement patterns, and coordination. By using gadgets that force you through a set motion, none of these latter qualities are improved.

HOOYA!

If you know very lean men or women who do only cardiovascular training, they're thin *not* because of their exercise but because they are naturally blessed with a fast metabolism and/or they eat a proper diet. For all the rest of us, cardio does little in the short term and can have negative effects in the long term.

HOOYA!

Low-intensity activity in the "fat-burning zone" does not build muscle, and it will cause muscle wasting if overused, which in turn *slows* your metabolism. High-intensity activity does build muscle, which *increases* your metabolism.

Many Nautilus-type machines are built for big men and are not ideally suited for women. Often, they begin movements in the most vulnerable position. Consider a pec deck or preacher curl. Both begin the movement with your isolated working muscles fully stretched. Then they force you through a fixed motion that you'll likely never use in the real world. This is especially hazardous under heavy loads. Because your body is not functioning naturally, as a cohesive whole, ineffective motor patterns are developed, making you more susceptible to injury.

The Myth of Spot Training and Low-Weight/High-Rep Effectiveness

Many women isolate muscles on machinery because they think that they can best reshape "problem" areas like abs or thighs or the butt through "spot training" with isolation exercises. Impossible. They also go for low weights and high reps on machines because they worry that strength training through low repetition of high-intensity movements will bulk them up in an unfeminine way. Won't happen. Some women I've talked to even think that any muscle they build through training can turn into flab if they don't keep working out. Oh, boy.

Let me address that last one right off the bat: Fat cells and muscle cells perform completely different and separate functions. One will never transform into the other. When someone becomes "soft" and overweight after being firm and lean, it is because their calorie input has exceeded their calorie output. This is usually due to 1) eating things to temporarily please your mind as opposed to pleasing your body and 2) a decreased metabolic rate from muscle loss caused by a lack of necessary stimulus—use it or lose it!

There's no magical transformation of muscle into fat, just a loss of muscle mass and an increase of body fat. Similarly, fat will never turn into muscle. When an overweight person becomes firm and lean, it is always the product of burning more calories than are being consumed and building new muscle.

Let me dispel the other rumors one at a time:

SPOT TRAINING, ISOLATION EXERCISES, AND TONING UP: THE THREE DEAD-END EXERCISE METHODS

Every time I'm fresh back from a few months abroad and standing in any American airport kiosk, I'm always astonished to see that magazine covers—both women's and men's—still boast some new crunch exercise that promises to make a six-pack magically pop out of your belly like a rabbit out of a hat.

Such proclamations are a load of bull and ought to be exiled to late-night infomercials where they belong: "Call now, and in four easy installments of $19.95 you, too, can climb into this gimmicky contraption and look like our smiling fitness models, who had never seen one of these ab-ominations before they stepped onto the set this morning."

Crunching away like the model in the magazine won't make your abs any flatter; using a ThighMaster will not make your inner thighs any leaner. If the backs of your upper arms seem a little flabby, cranking out triceps kickbacks with light dumbbells isn't the answer.

Fat loss simply cannot be isolated to a particular area of the body, because fat can only be lost over your whole body. To repeat: You can't specifically exercise it away from a chosen body part.

When you expend more calories (energy) than you consume, you create a deficit. In order to keep you moving, your body uses its own fat—through a series of chemical reactions that takes place throughout tissue all over your body—to cover the gap between consumed and expended energy. The areas of your body where those chemical reactions occur most can't be controlled, just as you cannot control where fat accumulates.

What *is* true is that the regions where you are genetically programmed to accumulate fat fastest—such as your hips, thighs, and butt—will likewise undergo the greatest proportional decreases in fat.

Fat loss and gain may be universal, but muscle growth, on the other hand, is confined to only those regions you work out. Still, let's be clear: The shape that your muscles take, as they change in size, is determined not by the specific exercises you do but by genetics. (Some body parts that we often think of as single muscles—such as your shoulders, thighs, or back—are actually muscle *groups*. The shapes of these muscle groups can be changed by emphasizing individual muscles within them.)

HOOYA!

Fat loss can't be isolated. The only way to tighten certain regions is to reduce fat on your entire body, which will in turn reduce fat in that region. Only then will the effort you're expending to, say, strengthen your triceps or firm up your thighs yield new curves and firmness in them.

Another way of saying this is that you can choose which body parts to make stronger, and that effort, in turn, will help your overall fat loss. So while doing exercises for your arms will do little to work the flab off them specifically, the effort will strengthen your arms and in turn help burn fat off your entire body, arms included.

Similarly, if you're looking for a firm backside, yes, you should develop your glutes. But unless you are burning fat off your entire body, increasing the muscle in your glutes will do little to firm up that region. Remember, your muscles will not look toned unless there is little fat masking them.

LOW REPS, HIGH WEIGHTS, BULGING MUSCLES, AND OTHER MISINFORMATION

Maybe you've been told that low-rep bodyweight strength training will bulk you up. Or, conversely, that working your muscles with small amounts of weight over and over and over again is the key to toning them and not building them. Not so. For starters, see what I said above about the myth of "toning" any one muscle.

The reality is that strength training my way will make you smaller, not bigger, because increasing lean muscle mass will burn up fat over your entire body. Yet still I hear it from women all over the world: "I don't want to get too muscular." Some have seen the initial results of strength training and then shied away in fear of becoming the next Ms. Olympia.

First off, in case you didn't already know, male and female professional bodybuilders competing at the highest levels (and most likely some of the bigger guys at your gym) all use steroids and other illegal substances. The human body—yours included—simply will not accrue that kind of muscle mass without serious drugs.

For men and women, some good initial gains in muscularity are common within the first few weeks, but after that your body adapts and growth slows down to a decent, stable level.

A woman making exceptional progress might gain 1.5 pounds of muscle per month, for the first three months. With a good diet, these muscular gains will be accompanied by a fat loss of six to eighteen pounds, depending on her condition. After that, women simply do not have the hormonal makeup to maintain that kind of gain in muscular size (and neither do men). So while the muscle you built will continue to help you shed more and more fat, because it's boosted your metabolism, body-weight strength training will not continue to increase the size of your muscles (beyond giving your body some new curves).

Overcoming the media-driven misconception and unfounded fear that strength training will build big bulky muscles is essential. Those men who strength-train without drugs celebrate every extra millimeter of muscle. That's because it's really hard to pack on muscle for us. And it's quite a bit tougher for females, who lack the testosterone that lets men do it. You simply can't and won't get bulky.

So what about the issue of reps?

Neither your body nor a particular muscle will become more defined by doing a high rather than a low amount of repetitions. High-rep "toning" workouts do little to improve muscle tone, because, again, they are effective at neither burning fat nor building muscle. This is largely because they develop only the weaker, slow-twitch muscle fibers.

> **HOOYA!**
>
> With a well-designed program, about 90 minutes or less of strength training a *week* is all that's needed for novices and many elite athletes alike.
>
> Any activities beyond this should be either light ones to aid recovery or sport-specific ones—for example, soccer practice if you play soccer. Working out more than is necessary only prolongs recovery and slows progress. Your muscles and your body change not during exercise but during rest. Let's not make this harder than it has to be. Train hard, but train smart. Leave yourself valuable time to recover instead of pushing yourself too hard.

While many men are all about stacking the barbell plates on at the cost of precision, women are often all about precision at the cost of challenge.

Again, only a muscle's size and the amount of fat over it determine how lean and defined it looks, period. For a lean physique, we need to do what most effectively builds muscle and burns fat. The answer: intense strength training in the 3-to-12-rep range and eating properly. Doing higher reps does not burn more calories than doing low reps. In fact, it burns less because it builds less fat-burning muscle.

The Myth of Male and Female Workout Needs

I hate to be the bearer of bad news, but the typical strength training that many women do is nearly useless. Going from machine to machine—using resistance that isn't very challenging—will yield limited results for the first couple of months at best, but, honestly, so will anything short of bed rest.

Men and women have different hormones and (usually) different fitness goals, but the best methods to achieve those different goals are the same.

Most women aren't looking to develop big arms but rather to firm and tone the entire body, especially their legs and bellies and glutes, which tend to be the hardest areas to maintain. The ironic thing is that you should do exactly the same thing to achieve this goal as men should to bulk up.

Since women don't have the hormonal makeup that allows men to get big muscles, most women simply won't achieve men's goals. Instead, they will achieve their own goals of getting a leaner, harder body.

While a woman's muscles won't get as big as a man's from strength training, the stimulus to make a woman's muscle bigger and stronger is identical to that of a man's: overload the muscle with progressively greater workloads.

Women too often take their arms along for the ride when they work out. Some women continually fail to understand that if they exercised their upper bodies as much as their lower, their tummies would just be that much flatter and their glutes that much tighter, because they would be increasing their overall lean muscle mass.

HOOYA!

There is an enormous difference in appearance between a thin female with muscle and a thin female without muscle. The latter often has the same body-fat percentage as someone quite a bit bigger, but due to the lack of any significant muscle mass she appears to be thinner. This is commonly referred to as "skinny fat," and it is often the result of weight loss through aerobic activity and calorie restriction only. Yet another reason why it pays not to worry about weight loss but instead to focus on body composition and performance.

As you age, without exercise your metabolism dips and your body becomes softer due to a loss of muscle. The average female loses five percent of her muscle per decade after the age of thirty. This causes an average weight gain of 2.2 pounds per year; it's generally agreed that inactive women over the age of forty lose muscle twice as fast as inactive men do.

But this weight-gain trend is halted and reversed by the calories required to keep just three pounds of extra muscle alive. This becomes more and more important as your age increases. Precisely because women don't have enough testosterone to retain muscle the way men do, the benefits of strength training are actually more important to women.

But it's not all about looking good. Effective strength training improves bone density (helping you avoid fractures and breaks), joint resilience, balance, coordination, flexibility, stability, strength, and cardiovascular endurance; this in turn lowers your risk of arthritis, osteoporosis (which affects women more than men), obesity, depression, back pain, insomnia, poor libido, poor posture, injury, and immobility, among other ailments. Gaining strength even lowers blood-sugar levels and cholesterol, reducing your risk for heart disease and type 2 diabetes.

Let's put it this way: Falls bring more people over the age of sixty-five to assisted-living facilities than anything else. As strength diminishes, so does stability, which increases your chances of falling while making you less able to deal with the impact.

Working out when you're young is the best prevention. But it's never too late. Improvements are possible at any age. Women in their seventies and eighties can still build important strength through bodyweight exercises.

Strength, more than any other factor—whether physical or financial—is essential to maintaining your quality of life as you age. Strength training is practical. Steady-state aerobic activity is not. Being strong is being able to move through life with ease.

2

Why Bodyweight Training Is the Key to Your Best Body Ever

There's a common misperception out there that bodyweight-exercise options are limited. Push-ups, Pull-ups, Sit-ups—and not much else. *Hmmmm* . . . Did I mention that there are 125 different exercises or variations in this book alone, with many more in *You Are Your Own Gym*?

Other people think it's impossible to work certain muscle groups with bodyweight exercises. Wrong again. Every single muscle group, and some you probably didn't know existed, can be worked without weights.

My bodyweight exercises use multi-joint movements, engaging many muscles at once, making them far more efficient than other types of exercises. With most fitness machines and weight-lifting exercises, you're sitting or lying down while isolating only certain muscles. This is extremely time-consuming if you're planning to work your whole body. There simply isn't a good reason for it unless you enjoy spending unnecessary time at a gym and getting mediocre results.

Isolation exercises also require that you spend time separately doing aerobic workouts, because using individual muscles doesn't create much of a demand for oxygen. However, movements that engage many large muscles and small stabilizing muscles at once require a great deal of energy. This in turn requires the heart to work much harder. The heart supports the muscles, and both should be challenged simultaneously, as they are in real-life situations.

Remember, form follows function. Functional bodyweight exercises are the best way to develop the body you want.

The Six Principles Behind My Program

The most widely used fitness programs today are fundamentally flawed and devoid of a well-thought-out structure. Honestly, just about any kind of exercise will bring some results for the first month or two. The true test comes afterward.

Mine was the first exercise program in history to combine bodyweight exercises with time-tested methods of structuring strength training. I then applied, tweaked, and enhanced the following six key principles in order to create the fastest possible changes in body composition for you.

1. CONSISTENCY AND REGULARITY

Most conventional strength-training programs split routines into body parts that are trained only once a week. This means that you perform the most effective, multi-joint movements once every seven days, if at all.

With my program, you'll focus on only the most effective movements and perform them three times a week. This means that you'll build more strength and burn more calories with less of your valuable time.

2. OVERLOAD

As you advance and your body adapts, you'll need greater amounts of stress to spur further progress. My program starts with short and easy workouts that progressively become harder. The correct application of stress at just the right time is a science I've perfected, and it'll keep you getting leaner and stronger.

3. RECOVERY

In the beginning, you'll need only two days to recover from a workout, because the stress applied was minimal. But as your body changes and adapts over time, you'll need to increase the stress, which will require a proportionate increase in recovery time. My variation in workout intensity and volume allows for greater recovery while preventing the loss of movement proficiency.

4. PROGRESSION

In order to provide you with exercises that challenge you appropriately, I've split all 125 of this book's exercises into five Movement Categories (Pulling, Squatting, In-line Pushing, Perpendicular Pushing, and Bending), which gradually progress from easiest to hardest. This allows you to methodically conquer even the toughest exercises.

5. VARIETY

Variety doesn't mean using different exercises every time you work out. Variety must be applied to intensity and volume.

I've created three cycles with varying volume and intensity that account precisely for your changing needs for stress and recovery. Each cycle is a four-week progression.

Cycle 1

This first cycle is designed for your ability to initially make workout-to-workout progress. You'll see a wide variety of exercise variations in this phase of training as you conquer new exercises.

Cycle 2

This cycle begins the week with a harder workout, uses a recovery workout at midweek, and offers an end-of-week workout that measures progress while getting you another good day of training. This cycle sets you up for weekly progress after workout-to-workout progress is no longer possible.

Cycle 3

Three hard workouts within the same week create residual fatigue that carries over into the following week. Then you'll have two low-volume workouts that allow for recovery without detraining. This cycle is designed for biweekly progress.

6. THERE IS NO ONE-SIZE-FITS-ALL

People's ability to recover varies depending on genetics, sleep, diet, environmental stress, and levels of advancement. These factors will determine how long each of the three cycles continues to be effective for you personally.

An experienced bodyweight athlete will not be able to maintain the workout-to-workout progress of Cycle 1 as long as a complete novice. Similarly, a more advanced bodyweight athlete will not be able to maintain the week-to-week progress of Cycle 2 as long as her less-trained counterpart. See page 46 for tips on finding the right time to shift from one cycle to the next. One size doesn't fit all—I'll help you find your fit!

Regardless of level of advancement, anyone unfamiliar with the training structure of this program should be able to make progress with each cycle for at least a month.

HOOYA!

You Only Get Good at What You Do

Using machines makes you good at, well, using machines. Not much else.

Our training must reflect the demands of the real world to be most effective. Bodyweight exercises teach us to function naturally, as a cohesive whole, as we do in everyday life.

Don't waste your time becoming proficient at using fitness machines. Instead, become proficient at using the one thing that you are never without: your body.

Staying Motivated

3

In a nationwide survey of nearly a thousand women from all fifty states, we found that "lack of motivation" was the second-biggest reason women do not work out (the first being "no time"—which my program conquers). Some said they needed a significant other to do it with them. Some said a group would motivate them. Some said they thrived on competition to spur them along. A few women actually stated that they would not work out unless someone gave them cold hard cash to do so. Well, while increased energy and focus in your business life is just one of the myriad dividends of my program, I'm not really here to show you the money, honey.

For almost everyone I know, *results* are the ultimate motivator. You start to see a change in your physique, and your effort and positive attitude gain momentum: Seeing is believing.

As you continue to train, you'll see the results—new lines, a new shape, the curves of growing muscles, a hardness you didn't have before. Your body will change. With consistency, you'll start to look better and you will always continue to.

If you follow my program, you *will* attain the figure you desire. How long it takes to get there, though, will depend on how far away you are. Consider the following real-world examples:

Ann was a pretty fit, 130-pound female at 20 percent body fat. After two months on my program, she replaced six pounds of fat with three pounds of muscle. So while she lost six pounds of fat, the scale told her she lost only three pounds total bodyweight, which was true. In two months, she changed her body-fat percentage from 20 percent to 15 percent. This overall change in bodyweight of only three pounds gave her a 25 percent reduction in body fat! All while *increasing* her metabolism with new muscle.

Ann's change in body composition was relatively easy yet significant. It improved her appearance, metabolism, athleticism, and her overall ability to make continued progress.

Now let's look at Mary. She weighed in at 230. She began my strength-training program, stuck to it for two months, stepped on the scale every day, and then became discouraged that she had lost only nine pounds after all that hard training. She now weighed 221 pounds, hardly where she wanted to be. And although the three pounds of muscle she gained were very real, she could hardly see them because, unlike Ann, she still had a lot of fat masking them. Her morale took a nosedive, and, before you know it, she succumbed to any excuse at all not to work out. She not only gained the weight back but continued her long, slow descent into morbid obesity.

Mary actually made better progress than the skinnier Ann, though of course it didn't show as much to the naked eye. What Mary didn't realize is that, while she lost fat, she also gained strength. It might not sound like much, but she made a significant change in body composition. She lost twelve pounds of fat and added three pounds of muscle. This increased her metabolism, setting her up for even greater success. If Mary continued to work out, this success would snowball: She'd accrue more muscle, be able to train more intensely, and thus burn more fat per week as time went on. It would get easier and easier.

And, no, Mary would not become a she-hulk! It's important to realize that the weight increase from muscle gain will slow significantly after these first three months of strength training, while the weight decrease from fat loss will only accelerate.

This is quite different from what most people do. Usually, people lose fat while also losing muscle. That may satisfy the need to see a smaller number on the scale, but it makes long-term success nearly unattainable.

For Mary, who has almost one hundred pounds to lose, it will take time. But it *will* happen. You can and will have the kind of body you want, but if you're far from your goal, you must be patient for the change to be real and lasting.

I know: *It sucks*. Waiting sucks. But it's simply *impossible* to magically undo ten years of neglect in two months. Nothing can do that for you. No pills, contraptions, or diets. With my program, you'll lose real fat, and you'll build real muscle to make sure it doesn't come back.

Remember, a pound of muscle takes up about half the space of a pound of fat. So if you lose three pounds of fat around your waist, that decrease will show much more than the slight increase in your muscles that leads to firmer triceps and legs.

Dealing with the Dreaded Scale and That Mirror, Mirror, on the Wall

As Ann and Mary's examples show, bathroom scales don't tell the whole story. Challenge yourself to stay off the scale for at least the first two months of training, and then look at the scale once a month afterward, maximum, or only if you must for some other reason. Otherwise, there's no need at all to look at the scale. It's neither going to show you what you want to see nor reflect the very real progress you're making.

Actually, I not only recommend you stay off your scale, I recommend trashing or donating it. A scale is an incredibly poor indicator of progress, especially in women, whose weight can rise and fall significantly due to water retention, with daily fluctuations of up to six pounds being possible.

A daily glance in the mirror is not going to be the best indicator of the ways in which your body composition is changing on this program, but consider taking a picture of yourself before you start and then another after two months of doing my program three times a week. I'll bet that, just like in those dramatic before-and-after infomercial photos, you'll be able to see the difference if you document it. Want to brag about your great progress? Send your before-and-after photos to me at YouAreYourOwnGym.com so that everyone can see your new physique! Use these photos to motivate yourself even more—paste your "before" photo on the blank page at the end of this book, then add the "after" in two short months.

Instead, make performance-related goals, not weight-related ones. Challenge yourself to move up through my exercise progressions as quickly as you can. You'll begin to look like an athlete once you start performing like one.

It's hard not to constantly obsess over appearance. But just as that dreaded scale is a bad indicator of progress, so, too, is the mirror. Looking in the mirror every day is something most of us can't avoid, and some people can use vanity—the desire to look better in that mirror—to their advantage; the mirror becomes a kind of taskmaster, a constant reminder to keep up the workouts. If that describes you, great. Use your mirror to motivate you.

But know, too, that mirrors can blind us to any real changes that occur over time, precisely because we look at ourselves every day. With my program and nutritional advice, your body most certainly will change week to week, month to month, but you're not going to notice any definitive change from one day to the next.

A better indicator of your progress is how your clothes fit. Over time, you'll start to see changes in them. Your shirts will be a little looser and your pants baggier, especially around the waist and hips. And whether they tell you or not, people around you will notice.

No More Excuses

Sometimes after a long day, lifting the remote is about all I seem to have strength for. It feels great to lie down on the couch, flip the tube on, and laugh with my favorite show. The Internet, Facebook, my cellphone—they are all such sweet temptations. My friends are at happy hour down the street, but I have to work out. . . . *Why?* I promise myself that I'll make up for it in the morning, but when morning comes around, the snooze button suddenly becomes man's greatest invention.

When it's time to exercise, don't ever forget that 1,001 excuses will rear their ugly heads every single day. Later will never be easier than now. You absolutely must shut out everything else. Turn your phone off. Forget about work, family, friends, and anything that can get in your way of achieving a better, healthier life. Don't worry: When you're done, you'll return to the world more energized and stronger than ever, ready to tackle just about anything. But right here, right now, this is *your time*. The world can wait.

While the troops I've trained face the immediate danger of bullets and bombs, we all face the long-term dangers of immobility and disease. My program can help protect people from both. But you must temporarily set aside your comfort and train, because you have made a decision to become a healthier person, one short workout at a time, and that is simply more important than any fatigue or stress that you might be dealing with. It's a small, immediate sacrifice for a better-looking, healthier you.

No more excuses! Don't skip a workout or promise yourself you'll do it later. *Skip one single workout and it can be very difficult to ever get started again.* I've seen it time and again: Quitting once makes it far more likely that you'll do it again. Likewise, every time you push the excuses aside, your resolve is strengthened. Your behavior *now* directly affects your behavior in the future. So EVOLVE: Earn Victory Over Life's Vast Excuses. Make winning a habit.

Put It in Writing

I want you to write down the daily excuses you come up with that prevent you from reaching your goals. Do it in two columns and see for yourself—goals and excuses side by side—how you too often obstruct your goals with your lame excuses.

Over time, after you see the results of my program, your excuses will fade. But in the beginning, rack them up! Write out as many as you can beside your goals before you work out each day. I've included several blank "Goals/Excuses" sheets at the end of this book—cut them out, use them, post them where you can see your goals (and make note of your lame excuses) every day! Only when you've conquered your worst excuses can your objectives become attainable.

The big things, the little things, and all the crap in the middle will always be there. Just remember, there are very few priorities in life that should come above your own health and beauty. Put yourself, not your excuses, in control.

What Happens When You Let Your Excuses Take Over

bad moods	low bone density
anxiety	arthritis
tension	immobility
boredom	heart disease
depression	diabetes
insomnia	colon cancer
poor libido	obesity
weakness	a second-rate life
back pain	

What Happens When You Take Control

lose fat	better balance
look better	better posture
feel better	better coordination
increased energy	better flexibility
a firmer body	better stability
less stress	better cardiovascular endurance
improved self-esteem	a leaner, stronger you!

Need more motivation? Here are seven ideas and actions that will help you jump over your hurdles.

1. YOU'VE ALREADY STARTED

Picking up this book may be the hardest part of my workout program. You've already made the decision to get into the best shape of your life.

The second-hardest part is getting started on your workout days. In one of the compounds we set up in Afghanistan, we built a small makeshift workout room that we affectionately called the "prison gym." When I was there recently, one of my Air Force buddies put it perfectly when he told me, "Once I'm going, I'm good. It's just getting myself to walk those thirty feet from my bed rack to the prison gym that's the hardest."

Get out of your seat and take that first step! It's easy sailing from there.

2. ENJOY THE JOURNEY

For a lot of people, exercise is *boooooring*. Well, when you're doing an hour or more of the same

HOOYA!

An Emergency Situation

Just as dozens of small excuses will rear their heads daily, occasionally real excuses will also arise: A debilitating injury that cannot be trained around. The last few months of pregnancy. The death of a loved one. They can happen to all of us. (Well, I guess I can't quite get pregnant yet, but you get the point.) Naturally, these are times when it is okay to put a pause on your training.

I must admit, though, that sometimes my training is what helps me meet life's greatest difficulties with strength. But that is a personal choice, and sometimes exercise becomes impossible due to severe emotional or physical stress. So take a breather. When you are ready again, the program will still be here for you.

One thing I would caution is not to wallow too long in the wake of these inevitable, life-changing events. As soon as you are in a mental and emotional place to fit exercise back into your days, you'll be best off doing so. Rebuilding your body can only help to rebuild your spirits.

thing every day, of course it's boring! Honestly, I'd rather sit at the DMV for an hour than spend that time in the fat-burning zone on an elliptical.

My program changes from day to day, week to week, month to month. You'll have fun conquering new movements rather than doing the same thing over and over.

If it's a nice day, take it outside. A blast of sun and fresh air can do wonders for the soul, not to mention your motivation.

"I go to exercise classes and used to go to a trainer, mostly because of the knowledge that I assume the instructor has."

—KELLY, 24, GRADUATE STUDENT, SPRINGFIELD, MISSOURI

For some people, a major obstacle to working out alone is the lack of confidence to correctly and effectively strength-train without an "expert" telling them how to. In my experience, the reality is that many gym trainers just throw random workouts together based on the handful of exercises they know and prefer. Many people don't realize most instructors' lack of expertise and the ease with which their personal-trainer certifications are acquired.

The reality is, if you follow the detailed illustrations and exercise descriptions in this book, you'll have a far greater understanding of the fundamentals than most trainers could give you. I'll show you exactly what basic exercises to focus on and how to make the slight adjustments for all their variations. I'll guide you through the subtle things that make these movements perfect, so you can continue to build on a solid foundation.

Regardless of where you exercise, since you're the boss now, crank the tunes as loud as you want, earphones or not. Heck, turn the tube on if there's a show you want to catch. Just be sure it doesn't distract you from devoting proper intensity to each of your sets.

Of course, the truly interesting thing to watch is *you*. You learning new movements. You becoming leaner and more athletic than ever before. And the real fun is not during the exercise but during the rest of the day. Feeling and looking better is simply more fun. My short workouts pay enormous dividends once each is over: Stress is washed away, your mind and body are revitalized, your self-esteem is lifted, and those feel-good endorphins explode through your body. There's nothing boring about that.

3. FIND YOUR TIME—THIS IS YOUR TIME

Setting a specific time to exercise each day helps most people, including me. Find a time—morning, lunch break, evening—and stick to it.

Don't ever think, "I'll wait and see if I have time," or "I'll try to squeeze it in later." That'll never happen. Make a date with yourself. Then hold yourself accountable. The great thing is that this set time is whenever works best for *your* schedule.

Your livelihood depends upon someone creating time for you to work. Biology has dictated time for us to sleep. Food, drink, and entertainment businesses have created all sorts of times for you to enjoy yourself. However, no one but you can or will create time for you to *work out*.

There will never be the "perfect" time and conditions to do a workout. You have to create them, just as we all create excuses, every day, every hour, every minute, not to work out.

4. LET ME HEAR YOU SAY IT

Every Monday morning, tell yourself, *out loud*, that you will do my workouts that week. Be specific. Tell yourself that you will work out on your chosen three days. For example, "I will complete this week's workouts on Monday, Wednesday, and Friday."

It sounds funny, but studies have shown that a simple declaration like this can dramatically increase physical activity. It makes you consciously aware of your plans and encourages you to realize them.

5. YOU HAVE YOUR OWN FULL BODY FITNESS CENTER

Although you can do my workouts anywhere you find yourself in the world, it helps to have one space you use regularly. Whether it's your living room, bedroom, office, garage, or garden, find the place where it's best and most convenient to do the exercises in my program. For a few minutes each day, make it your very own full-body fitness center. Getting to know a single space well and the everyday things you can use to work out within it—a chair, desk, or doorway, for example—will make it easier to accomplish each exercise.

6. JUST IMAGINE

Use the mirror at your own risk, but don't stop *imagining* what you want to look like. Visualizing your goals is the first step toward them.

If you want to be leaner, with a smaller waist, toned arms and legs, and a butt firm enough to bounce quarters off, then you should imagine exactly how that is going to look and feel, with as much detail as possible.

Make yourself believe, and believe in yourself. Visualize the rewards that you will reap from your training, and make them a reality.

HOOYA!

Tear Down This Wall

Fat is a very real physical barrier you—and you alone—can either construct or tear down between yourself and a loved one. A lack of physical fitness is one of the greatest barriers to intimacy on the planet. You're literally putting on layers (of fat), constructing walls that not only hide you from the world but distance you from your partner. On the other hand, a healthy body is the greatest stimulation that exists.

HOOYA!

Go Solo

Now, don't get me wrong: Doing my program with a partner, or a group, is great. I love working out with other men or women in the Special Operations community or with my girlfriend. But you should never, not ever, *depend* on a partner in order to exercise. That becomes just another crutch, an excuse to not work out when they're not around. Drop the crutches. There should be no one to motivate you and hold you accountable other than yourself. A bodyweight athlete should never depend on anyone but herself. Your health is not a team sport. Your life is yours. And only you can excel at it.

"I work out alone because no one knows my body better than I do. Hey, I'm the only one living in it!"

—JENNIFER, 41, HEDGE-FUND LAWYER, NEW YORK CITY

"Working out is a great time to enjoy being alone. And it's productive. My job is people-to-people all day long, whether face-to-face or by phone. It's highly stimulating, so working out by myself gives me that sense of solace. You can call it recharge time."

—CHRIS, 63, WRITER, NEW ORLEANS, LOUISIANA

7. SCORE A GOAL

Remember, vanity will get you only so far.

Know why you're working out, and make your reasons true to you. Write them out on a piece of paper and post them wherever you will see them most: the bathroom mirror, the fridge, or your workout space. This will remind you every day why you are exercising. And fully accept that these goals are a *reality*. They will happen—as long as you get started every day you're supposed to work out.

It's certainly okay to focus on things like slimming your thighs, looking good in a new dress, putting the best you forward in a new romance, a new job, a new project, or even just looking better than your girlfriends. But you need to also ask yourself why exercise is a positive aspect of your life, how it will genuinely improve you and the world around you. These goals will provide sources of instant, continual, and meaningful inspiration to drive you on. Envision a better future, and you'll become increasingly motivated to achieve it.

PART II

The *Body by You* Program

4

Your Training Schedule

You'll find all the exercises in this book organized by Movement Categories: Pulling, Squatting, In-line Pushing, Perpendicular Pushing, and Bending. Within these categories, exercises progress gradually from easiest to hardest. Difficulty isn't adjusted by adding a weight (as on a machine or with free weights) but rather by changing the intensity of movements through leverage, pauses, and single- or double-limb engagement.

LEVERAGE

Let's take the Push-up. By elevating your hands on a surface, such as a countertop, a Push-up becomes relatively easy. By placing your hands on incrementally lower surfaces, the exercise becomes gradually more difficult, until the user ends up with her hands on the ground and her feet elevated.

PAUSES

An exercise becomes harder when you add short pauses at the most difficult portion of a movement. Pausing for two seconds at the bottom of a Squat makes it more difficult.

HOOYA!

The *Body by You* program takes the guesswork out of training. You'll know exactly what exercises to start with, how they're executed, and when to move on to harder exercises. As I was taught in the military, "You need a system and a plan. That's when you're dangerous!" You'll find yourself quickly conquering previously unreachable exercises and goals. The days of self-consciously moving between random machines with uncertainty are over.

TWO-LIMB TO SINGLE-LIMB

Movements can be made harder by switching from a two-limb movement to a single-limb movement. A Squat can be made harder by switching to an assisted One-legged Squat.

In Chapter 6, you'll find all the exercises, and their descriptions, organized by Movement Categories. Each exercise is numbered accordingly, and those are the numbers you will be plugging into your workout schedule. But before getting into all the exercises themselves, right now I want to introduce you to that schedule and the workout cycles.

The Five Components of Your Schedule

There are five simple components of your training: days, the Movement Categories, sets and reps, the exercises themselves, and intervals. At first glance, the workout charts may seem a little complex, but they're actually easy to understand. Let me break it down:

1. TRAINING DAYS

You will always train three days a week, with one day of rest between workouts. How you decide to split up your training days is completely up to you. I like to train on Monday, Wednesday, and Friday.

When you are looking at a chart of your training schedule, the far-left column displays which day you are on.

EXAMPLE:

DAY	MOVEMENT CATEGORY	SETS AND REPS	EXERCISE NUMBER	INTERVAL
Day 1	Pulling	2 x 12	3	2 minutes
	Squatting	2 x 12	5	3 minutes
	In-line Pushing	2 x 12	5	2 minutes
	Bending	2 x 12	5	3 minutes

2. MOVEMENT CATEGORIES

Remember that there are five Movement Categories in my workouts: Pulling, Squatting, In-line Pushing, Perpendicular Pushing, and Bending. On your schedule, the column to the right of the training day will tell you which Movement Categories to use and in what order.

EXAMPLE:

DAY	MOVEMENT CATEGORY	SETS AND REPS	EXERCISE NUMBER	INTERVAL
Day 1	Pulling	2 x 12	3	2 minutes
	Squatting	2 x 12	5	3 minutes
	In-line Pushing	2 x 12	5	2 minutes
	Bending	2 x 12	5	3 minutes

3. SETS AND REPS

The column to the right of the Movement Categories will tell you how many sets and repetitions to do.

One complete movement of an exercise is a repetition or "rep." A "set" is a series of repetitions done back-to-back.

The number of sets is displayed first, followed by a multiplication sign, and then the number of reps to perform for each set: 2 x 12 = two sets of twelve repetitions. That means you will do 12 reps, rest, and then finish with the second set of 12 reps.

EXAMPLE:

DAY	MOVEMENT CATEGORY	SETS AND REPS	EXERCISE NUMBER	INTERVAL
Day 1	Pulling	2 x 12	3	2 minutes
	Squatting	2 x 12	5	3 minutes
	In-line Pushing	2 x 12	5	2 minutes
	Bending	2 x 12	5	3 minutes

4. EXERCISES

Here's where you might need to pay a little more attention. The schedule will *not* tell you which specific exercises to use. Instead, under the "Exercise" column, you will input the numbers of the exercises appropriate for you from each Movement Category. The first two workouts of the program will be evaluations and will reveal to you which exercises are appropriate.

EXAMPLE OF WHAT YOU MIGHT WRITE IN:

DAY	MOVEMENT CATEGORY	SETS AND REPS	EXERCISE NUMBER	INTERVAL
Day 1	Pulling	2 x 12	3	2 minutes
	Squatting	2 x 12	5	3 minutes
	In-line Pushing	2 x 12	5	2 minutes
	Bending	2 x 12	5	3 minutes

5. INTERVALS

The far-right column tells you the interval duration for each Movement Category. An interval is the amount of time allotted for each set.

So, in the schedule below, you will start exercising as soon as the time for the interval begins, attempt to do the prescribed number of repetitions, and then rest until the time for that interval has elapsed, at which point you will begin the next set. On a 2-minute interval, if the first Pulling set takes you one minute to complete, then you have another minute to rest before the second set begins. Assuming the second set also takes you one minute, you have another minute of rest before moving on to the next Movement Category and your third set.

EXAMPLE:

DAY	MOVEMENT CATEGORY	SETS AND REPS	EXERCISE NUMBER	INTERVAL
Day 1	Pulling	2 x 12	3	2 minutes
	Squatting	2 x 12	5	3 minutes
	In-line Pushing	2 x 12	5	2 minutes
	Bending	2 x 12	5	3 minutes

The second Movement Category will be Squatting, which has a 3-minute interval. You do one set, then rest for the remainder of the 3 minutes. For example, if that set takes you 45 seconds, you rest for 2 minutes and 15 seconds, then do your second and last set of Squatting.

Then you move on to In-line Pushing: 2 sets at 2-minute intervals.

And last you'll do Bending: 2 sets at 3-minute intervals.

It's really pretty simple. All you need to do is pay attention to when to start each set. If you use the timer on your cellphone, for example, you'll begin Pulling at 0:00 and 2:00, Squatting at 4:00 and 7:00, Pushing at 10:00 and 12:00, and Bending at 14:00 and 17:00.

Similarly, if you go by a watch or clock, choose a time to begin, say 12:10. Do your first set, rest, then start your second set at 12:12 . . . and finish with your last set of Bending at 12:27.

It takes only about 18 minutes, and then you're done for the day!

Making Progress

Anytime you are able to do *all* prescribed reps in any particular Movement Category (with good form!), you're ready to upgrade to the next exercise. Just place an up arrow next to the current exercise number—the one you kicked butt on—so that you'll know to upgrade when that Movement Category is done again.

The sample training day below calls for 2 sets of 12 reps (2 x 12) in all Movement Categories.

For Pulling, if you do both sets of 12 reps with good form using exercise #3, you will place an up arrow next to the 3 after completing the second set. This is your indicator to upgrade to exercise #4 the next time you do a Pulling movement.

Then you'll continue to use exercise #4 until you can do all prescribed reps with good form, at which point you will upgrade once again.

EXAMPLE:

DAY	MOVEMENT CATEGORY	SETS AND REPS	EXERCISE NUMBER	INTERVAL
Day 1	Pulling	2 x 12	3 ↑	2 minutes
	Squatting	2 x 12	5	3 minutes
	In-line Pushing	2 x 12	5	2 minutes
	Bending	2 x 12	5	3 minutes

5

Getting Started

Your first goal on my program will be to find the most difficult exercise that you can accomplish within each Movement Category for 12 reps. This is your initial evaluation. Once you know where to start, you can begin your first 4-week cycle.

For each Movement Category listed on the schedule on page 37, attempt to perform 12 repetitions of the first exercise, with good form.

If you are successful, jump to exercise #3 and attempt another 12 reps. Continue to attempt 12 reps with the odd-numbered exercises until you cannot complete all 12 reps with good form.

The exercise that you will begin Cycle 1 with, for each Movement Category, is the one that you last completed successfully for 12 reps.

Example:

For Pulling, if you successfully did 12 reps of exercise #1 but then failed to complete all 12 reps of exercise #3, you would use exercise #1 on your first day of training.

For Squatting, if you successfully did 12 reps of exercises #1, 3, and 5 but your form got sloppy on exercise #7, then you would use exercise #5.

The evaluation for a particular Movement Category is over when your form begins to break down or you hit muscle failure. It's most likely that, as a beginner, your form will deteriorate before you reach muscle failure.

This could be due to a lack of balance, flexibility, strength, or generally being a little clumsy, like I am sometimes.

Rest at least a minute between exercises. There is no time limit. Don't feel rushed if you need to stop to look at exercise descriptions. And don't forget to warm up first.

HOOYA!

The Proper Warm-up

Conventional "static" stretching is insufficient and ill-suited for a real warm-up. Instead, here's how I would like you to ease into even the toughest workouts without wasted time or effort.

If you are using exercises #1 through 5 in any of the Movement Categories during your workout, you'll simply march in place for 1½ minutes, rest for 30 seconds, and then repeat before beginning the workout.

Everyone will use this warm-up for the initial evaluations.

Once you are using the sixth exercise or higher in each Movement Category, perform 6 reps of the first exercise in each of the following Movement Categories back-to-back:

1. Pulling (The first exercise being Let Me Ins with legs slightly bent, page 51)
2. Squatting (Therapy Sumo Squats, page 65)
3. Perpendicular Pushing (Push-ups with hands elevated sternum height, page 88)
4. Bending (Good Mornings, page 99)

Take a short breather and do 2 more rotations. After 3 rotations, you're ready to begin the main body of the workout. This shouldn't take more than 5 minutes. As you advance, or if you're already advanced, you can pick harder exercises for your warm-ups.

On Your Mark, Get Set, Go!

Okay. As we say in the military, you're "cleared hot" for the "destroy mission." Your targets? Pudgy and Feeble. It's time to do some work! Use the following schedule for your initial evaluations.

INITIAL EVALUATIONS

DAY	MOVEMENT CATEGORY	SETS AND REPS	EXERCISE NUMBER THAT YOU LAST COMPLETED WITH GOOD FORM:
Eval Day 1	Pulling	12 reps with odd-numbered exercises	
	Squatting	12 reps with odd-numbered exercises	
	Perp Pushing	12 reps with odd-numbered exercises	
Eval Day 2	In-line Pushing	12 reps with odd-numbered exercises	
	Bending	12 reps with odd-numbered exercises	

Cycle 1

Now you know with which exercises you should start your initial cycle. Use the following schedule to keep track of your first four weeks of effort.

CYCLE 1: WEEK 1

DAY	MOVEMENT CATEGORY	SETS AND REPS	EXERCISE NUMBER	INTERVAL
Day 1	Pulling	2 x 12		2 minutes
	Squatting	2 x 12		3 minutes
	In-line Pushing	2 x 12		2 minutes
	Bending	2 x 12		3 minutes
Day 2	Pulling	2 x 12		2 minutes
	Squatting	2 x 12		3 minutes
	Perp Pushing	2 x 12		2 minutes
	Bending	2 x 12		3 minutes
Day 3	Pulling	2 x 12		2 minutes
	Squatting	2 x 12		3 minutes
	In-line Pushing	2 x 12		2 minutes
	Bending	2 x 12		3 minutes

CYCLE 1: WEEK 2

DAY	MOVEMENT CATEGORY	SETS AND REPS	EXERCISE NUMBER	INTERVAL
Day 1	Pulling	2 x 12		2 minutes
	Squatting	2 x 12		3 minutes
	Perp Pushing	2 x 12		2 minutes
	Bending	2 x 12		3 minutes
Day 2	Pulling	2 x 12		2 minutes
	Squatting	2 x 12		3 minutes
	In-line Pushing	2 x 12		2 minutes
	Bending	2 x 12		3 minutes
Day 3	Pulling	2 x 12		2 minutes
	Squatting	2 x 12		3 minutes
	Perp Pushing	2 x 12		2 minutes
	Bending	2 x 12		3 minutes

↑ Place an up arrow next to any exercise that you're ready to upgrade!

CYCLE 1: WEEK 3

DAY	MOVEMENT CATEGORY	SETS AND REPS	EXERCISE NUMBER	INTERVAL
Day 1	Pulling	3 x 10		2 minutes
	Squatting	3 x 10		3 minutes
	In-line Pushing	3 x 10		2 minutes
	Bending	3 x 10		3 minutes
Day 2	Pulling	3 x 10		2 minutes
	Squatting	3 x 10		3 minutes
	Perp Pushing	3 x 10		2 minutes
	Bending	3 x 10		3 minutes
Day 3	Pulling	3 x 10		2 minutes
	Squatting	3 x 10		3 minutes
	In-line Pushing	3 x 10		2 minutes
	Bending	3 x 10		3 minutes

CYCLE 1: WEEK 4

DAY	MOVEMENT CATEGORY	SETS AND REPS	EXERCISE NUMBER	INTERVAL
Day 1	Pulling	3 x 10		2 minutes
	Squatting	3 x 10		3 minutes
	Perp Pushing	3 x 10		2 minutes
	Bending	3 x 10		3 minutes
Day 2	Pulling	3 x 10		2 minutes
	Squatting	3 x 10		3 minutes
	In-line Pushing	3 x 10		2 minutes
	Bending	3 x 10		3 minutes
Day 3	Pulling	3 x 10		2 minutes
	Squatting	3 x 10		3 minutes
	Perp Pushing	3 x 10		2 minutes
	Bending	3 x 10		3 minutes

↑ Place an up arrow next to any exercise that you're ready to upgrade!

Cycle 2

Same instructions as for Cycle 1, except we're adding "Dynamic Efforts."

The emphasis for these workouts is perfect technique and *fast*, powerful contractions, executing the concentric (upward) movements as fast as humanly possible. That's the positive portion of the movement, the part where you're doing either the pushing or pulling. You're always moving upward during this part. For example, with a Push-up, it's when you are pushing your body up. With a Pull-up, it's when you're pulling your body up. With a warrior, it's when you're moving your upper body upward.

Execute these concentric movements as fast as you can, not as fast as you can't! Maximum concentric speed, with perfect form, is what makes these workouts effective.

The negative portions of the exercises remain the same, and you'll exclude all pauses.

Your ability to engage motor neurons and in turn recruit more muscle fibers will develop with practice. As this ability evolves, dynamic efforts will require more recovery and make the relatively easy second training day of the week more necessary.

Perform each dynamic-effort set on a 1-minute interval. You'll do 10 sets of only 3 repetitions with each exercise. That's 10 minutes for each exercise.

KEEPING YOURSELF ACCOUNTABLE

For each Movement Category, write down how many reps you did of the exercise that you were *unable* to complete for 12 reps during the initial evaluation. Then post those exercises—the ones that were a bit too tough—and how many reps you managed on the "Goals and Progress" forum at YouAreYourOwnGym.com.

This is also the place to post your goals if you want to keep yourself accountable. After 2 months, I want you to revisit those exercises—the ones you initially couldn't do for 12 reps—doing as many reps as you can with each. Then add those numbers to your original post. You'll be amazed!

MAKING PROGRESS

For Cycle 2, you will upgrade when you can do 3 sets of 9 reps with an exercise, which is measured only on Day 3 of each week. This cycle measures progress on a weekly basis rather than workout-to-workout. You should only have up arrows on Day 3 of each week!

CYCLE 2: WEEK 1

DAY	MOVEMENT CATEGORY	SETS AND REPS	EXERCISE NUMBER	INTERVAL
Day 1 Dynamic Efforts	Pulling	10 x 3		1 minute
	Squatting	10 x 3		1 minute
	Perp Pushing	10 x 3		1 minute
	Bending	10 x 3		1 minute
Day 2	Pulling	2 x 7		2 minutes
	Squatting	2 x 7		3 minutes
	In-line Pushing	2 x 7		2 minutes
	Bending	2 x 7		3 minutes
Day 3	Pulling	3 x 9		2 minutes
	Squatting	3 x 9		3 minutes
	Perp Pushing	3 x 9		2 minutes
	Bending	3 x 9		3 minutes

CYCLE 2: WEEK 2

DAY	MOVEMENT CATEGORY	SETS AND REPS	EXERCISE NUMBER	INTERVAL
Day 1 Dynamic Efforts	Pulling	10 x 3		1 minute
	Squatting	10 x 3		1 minute
	In-line Pushing	10 x 3		1 minute
	Bending	10 x 3		1 minute
Day 2	Pulling	2 x 7		2 minutes
	Squatting	2 x 7		3 minutes
	Perp Pushing	2 x 7		2 minutes
	Bending	2 x 7		3 minutes
Day 3	Pulling	3 x 9		2 minutes
	Squatting	3 x 9		3 minutes
	In-line Pushing	3 x 9		2 minutes
	Bending	3 x 9		3 minutes

↑ Place an up arrow next to any exercise that you're ready to upgrade!

CYCLE 2: WEEK 3

DAY	MOVEMENT CATEGORY	SETS AND REPS	EXERCISE NUMBER	INTERVAL
Day 1 Dynamic Efforts	Pulling	10 x 3		1 minute
	Squatting	10 x 3		1 minute
	Perp Pushing	10 x 3		1 minute
	Bending	10 x 3		1 minute
Day 2	Pulling	2 x 7		2 minutes
	Squatting	2 x 7		3 minutes
	In-line Pushing	2 x 7		2 minutes
	Bending	2 x 7		3 minutes
Day 3	Pulling	3 x 9		2 minutes
	Squatting	3 x 9		3 minutes
	Perp Pushing	3 x 9		2 minutes
	Bending	3 x 9		3 minutes

CYCLE 2: WEEK 4

DAY	MOVEMENT CATEGORY	SETS AND REPS	EXERCISE NUMBER	INTERVAL
Day 1 Dynamic Efforts	Pulling	10 x 3		1 minute
	Squatting	10 x 3		1 minute
	In-line Pushing	10 x 3		1 minute
	Bending	10 x 3		1 minute
Day 2	Pulling	2 x 7		2 minutes
	Squatting	2 x 7		3 minutes
	Perp Pushing	2 x 7		2 minutes
	Bending	2 x 7		3 minutes
Day 3	Pulling	3 x 9		2 minutes
	Squatting	3 x 9		3 minutes
	In-line Pushing	3 x 9		2 minutes
	Bending	3 x 9		3 minutes

↑ Place an up arrow next to any exercise
that you're ready to upgrade!

Cycle 3

In addition to the workouts from your first two cycles, you're now going to add one new workout called a "3-rep pyramid," a fantastic confidence builder that lets you sample upcoming exercises in a lower-rep range.

You will perform 3 sets of 3 repetitions per Movement Category, at the intervals specified on the schedule.

For this workout, you will *not* use the same exercise for each set of a Movement Category. The first set will be with your current exercise—the one that you could do for 3 sets of 9 reps during Cycle 2. The second set will be the exercise that is one step harder than your current exercise. The third set will be with the exercise that is two steps higher than your current exercise.

Example: If your current movement for Pulling is exercise #12, you will use exercise #12 for set 1, exercise #13 for set 2, and exercise #14 for set 3.

MAKING PROGRESS

In Cycle 3, you will upgrade when you can do 3 x 8 with an exercise, which is only measured every other week on Day 3. You should only have up arrows on Day 3 of weeks 2 and 4!

CYCLE 3: WEEK 1

DAY	MOVEMENT CATEGORY	SETS AND REPS	EXERCISE NUMBER	INTERVAL
Day 1 Dynamic Efforts	Pulling	10 x 3		1 minute
	Squatting	10 x 3		1 minute
	Perp Pushing	10 x 3		1 minute
	Bending	10 x 3		1 minute
Day 2	Pulling	4 x 6		2 minutes
	Squatting	4 x 6		3 minutes
	In-line Pushing	4 x 6		2 minutes
	Bending	4 x 6		3 minutes
Day 3	Pulling	3 x 7		2 minutes
	Squatting	3 x 7		3 minutes
	Perp Pushing	3 x 7		2 minutes
	Bending	3 x 7		3 minutes

CYCLE 3: WEEK 2

DAY	MOVEMENT CATEGORY	SETS AND REPS	EXERCISE NUMBER	INTERVAL
Day 1	Pulling	2 x 8		2 minutes
	Squatting	2 x 8		3 minutes
	In-line Pushing	2 x 8		2 minutes
	Bending	2 x 8		3 minutes
Day 2 3-Rep Pyramid	Pulling	3 x 3		2 minutes
	Squatting	3 x 3		3 minutes
	Perp Pushing	3 x 3		2 minutes
	Bending	3 x 3		3 minutes
Day 3	Pulling	3 x 8		2 minutes
	Squatting	3 x 8		3 minutes
	In-line Pushing	3 x 8		2 minutes
	Bending	3 x 8		3 minutes

↑ Place an up arrow next to any exercise
that you're ready to upgrade!

CYCLE 3: WEEK 3

DAY	MOVEMENT CATEGORY	SETS AND REPS	EXERCISE NUMBER	INTERVAL
Day 1 Dynamic Efforts	Pulling	10 x 3		1 minute
	Squatting	10 x 3		1 minute
	Perp Pushing	10 x 3		1 minute
	Bending	10 x 3		1 minute
Day 2	Pulling	4 x 6		2 minutes
	Squatting	4 x 6		3 minutes
	In-line Pushing	4 x 6		2 minutes
	Bending	4 x 6		3 minutes
Day 3	Pulling	3 x 7		2 minutes
	Squatting	3 x 7		3 minutes
	Perp Pushing	3 x 7		2 minutes
	Bending	3 x 7		3 minutes

CYCLE 3: WEEK 4

DAY	MOVEMENT CATEGORY	SETS AND REPS	EXERCISE NUMBER	INTERVAL
Day 1	Pulling	2 x 8		2 minutes
	Squatting	2 x 8		3 minutes
	In-line Pushing	2 x 8		2 minutes
	Bending	2 x 8		3 minutes
Day 2 3-Rep Pyramid	Pulling	3 x 3		2 minutes
	Squatting	3 x 3		3 minutes
	Perp Pushing	3 x 3		2 minutes
	Bending	3 x 3		3 minutes
Day 3	Pulling	3 x 8		2 minutes
	Squatting	3 x 8		3 minutes
	In-line Pushing	3 x 8		2 minutes
	Bending	3 x 8		3 minutes

↑ Place an up arrow next to any exercise that you're ready to upgrade!

Finding the right time to shift from one cycle to another ensures that the important principles of overload and recovery are applied properly. Use the following guidelines to help you find the right time to switch cycles:

Cycle 1

Repeat the last two weeks of this cycle until progress is halted for 3 consecutive workouts and you fail to upgrade in any Movement Category.

Cycle 2

Repeat this cycle until you fail to upgrade in any of the Movement Categories 2 weeks in a row.

Cycle 3

Repeat this cycle until you fail to make progress for an entire month. Thereafter, I recommend switching to the program in *You Are Your Own Gym* or adjusting the intensity and volume of Cycle 3 to suit your specific needs.

6

The Movement Categories, Progressions, and Exercises

T he 125 exercises I offer you here are separated into five Movement Categories: Pulling, Squatting, In-line Pushing, Perpendicular Pushing, and Bending. Each of the Movement Categories contains twenty-five exercises listed and described in order from easiest to hardest, #1 being the easiest and #25 the most difficult.

Top Tips

At the beginning of each Movement Category, you'll find top tips: expert advice that applies to all the exercises within that category.

EXERCISES AND VARIATIONS

Since each of the five Movement Categories gradually progresses from the easiest exercise to the hardest, you'll often find an original exercise appearing several times with only slight variations, usually with the addition of a one- or two-second pause. To keep you from reading the same material over and over, I mention the differences in variations only after giving the full, original exercise description. Those familiar with *You Are Your Own Gym* may recognize the names of a few of these exercises, though here I've tweaked those movements in order to perfect the progressions.

TAKE IT DOWN OR KICK IT UP

At the end of most exercise descriptions, you'll find *Need to take it down a notch?* This is a way to make the exercise just a little bit easier. It's useful if you find a jump from one exercise to another too difficult.

The last exercise of each Movement Category has a *Ready to kick it up a notch?* This explains how to progress after you've conquered the last movement.

PAUSES

We'll use 1- and 2-second pauses to increase the intensity of some movements. Don't cheat yourself. It can be very tempting to cut pauses short. A pause shouldn't begin until you are at a complete stop. The movement should begin again only after you are done counting out the pause.

To help accurately time each pause, say the duration of the pause during it.

For 1-second pauses, you'll say, "One-second pause," as soon as the pause begins. After you complete the count, you finish the repetition.

For 2-second pauses, you'll say, "One-second pause, two-second pause."

You don't need to count out loud, just make sure you're not rushing the count.

If you can't finish a set with the full pauses, you can shorten or remove pauses toward the end of a set to get those couple of extra reps. But don't move on to the next exercise until all reps are done using the prescribed pauses and, of course, good form.

HOUSEHOLD EQUIPMENT

For the exercises that require a prop, I mention appropriate common household items in the descriptions. But, remember, the most important thing when exercising is *not* your form, intensity, or breathing. It is your safety.

If you choose to exercise using surfaces such as a table, chairs, door, staircase, or anything else, make 100 percent sure they are stable, secure, and strong enough to support *all* of your weight.

If you're uncomfortable using such items or would just prefer something more convenient, go to YouAreYourOwnGym.com for information about the Bodyweight Bar. It easily installs in any doorway and allows you to do every single exercise in this book without the use of anything else.

Pulling Exercises

All Pulling movements work your entire back—lats, spinal erectors, rhomboids—as well as your biceps, forearms, rear deltoids, and core.

Top Tip

For all Pulling exercises, get a good stretch around your shoulder blades at the bottom of each repetition, with arms fully extended. Then squeeze your shoulder blades together as you begin each rep.

HOOYA!

Rep Speed

In my program, the negative portion of any movement (when your body is moving *downward*) should always take about 2 seconds. It's the concentric portion (when your body is moving *upward*) that should change slightly over time.

For unfamiliar exercises and warm-ups, you should begin with relatively slow contractions, lasting about 2 seconds on the way up, emphasizing control and technique. Once you're warmed up and proficient at a movement, start working on faster contractions in order to recruit as many muscle fibers as possible. Try to make them less than a second—for example, 2 seconds on the way down, less than 1 second on the way up. In this case, faster is better. Just remember to perform exercises as fast as you can, not as fast as you can't!

PULLING EXERCISES IN ORDER OF DIFFICULTY:

1. Let Me Ins with legs slightly bent
2. Let Me Ins with legs slightly bent and 2-second pauses
3. Let Me Ins
4. Let Me Ins with 2-second pauses
5. One-arm Let Me Ins with knees slightly bent
6. One-arm Let Me Ins with knees slightly bent and 2-second pauses
7. One-arm Let Me Ins
8. One-arm Let Me Ins with 2-second pauses
9. Let Me Ups with knees bent 90 degrees
10. Let Me Ups with knees bent 90 degrees and 1-second pauses
11. Let Me Ups with knees bent 90 degrees and 2-second pauses
12. Let Me Ups with knees slightly bent
13. Let Me Ups with knees slightly bent and 1-second pauses
14. Let Me Ups with knees slightly bent and 2-second pauses
15. Let Me Ups with legs straight
16. Let Me Ups with legs straight and 1-second pauses
17. Let Me Ups with legs straight and 2-second pauses
18. Let Me Ups with feet elevated
19. Assisted Pull-ups
20. Assisted Pull-ups with 2-second unassisted negative
21. Assisted Pull-ups with 3-second unassisted negative
22. Assisted Pull-ups with 4-second unassisted negative
23. Assisted Pull-ups with 3-second unassisted negative and 1-second pauses
24. Assisted Pull-ups with 4-second unassisted negative and 1-second pauses
25. Pull-ups

1. Let Me Ins with legs slightly bent

Hold a towel in front of the outside
edge of an open, sturdy door, just
above the doorknobs, so that the
door's edge runs down the middle
of the towel. Then wrap each end
of the towel over the top of the
doorknobs and bring the ends
underneath back toward you. (You

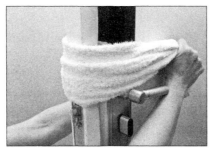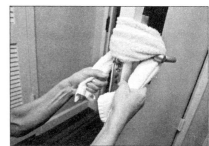

can also place a short thick rope or towel around any sturdy
pole—horizontal or vertical—at waist height for this purpose.)

Hold each end of the towel a couple of inches from the doorknobs or
handles.

Place your feet on either side of the
door, pressing the door between them.
Your feet should be directly below the
doorknobs, so that you're straddling the
door. Be sure that you have good
traction with the floor.

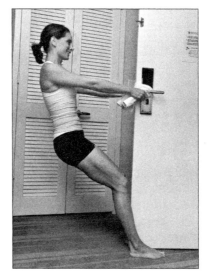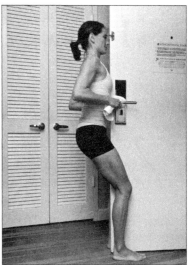

Lean back until your arms are fully
extended. Bend your knees 45 degrees,
keeping your back straight.

With your legs slightly bent and your
feet flat on the ground, pull your chest
all the way to your hands, really
squeezing the shoulder blades together.

Return to the starting position in a
controlled motion.

Need to take it down a notch?

Move your feet back slightly. As you develop more strength, move your
feet forward. Don't progress to the next movement until you're doing this
exercise with your feet under the doorknobs.

WATCH the workout—
SCAN here

2. Let Me Ins with legs slightly bent and 2-second pauses

Once your hands are touching your upper torso, hold yourself there for 2 seconds, squeezing your shoulder blades together.

3. Let Me Ins

This exercise is just like Let Me Ins with legs slightly bent, except your knees will remain bent 90 degrees, so that your thighs are parallel to the ground.

Be sure to keep your toes down on the ground. Only your ankles and your arms should move throughout this exercise. Your legs should always remain bent at 90 degrees.

It's common for people to feel their legs fatigue during this exercise. Like all bodyweight exercises, Let Me Ins work many muscles at once. Static strength increases very quickly, so it shouldn't be an issue for long.

Need to take It down a notch?
Straighten your legs slightly.

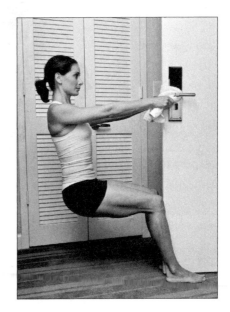

4. Let Me Ins with 2-second pauses

Once your hands are touching your upper torso, hold for 2 seconds, squeezing your shoulder blades together.

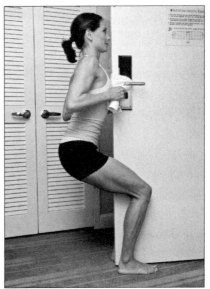

5. One-arm Let Me Ins with knees slightly bent

Start by fastening a reliable belt onto itself, so it forms a loop. Place the belt around one of the doorknobs or handles and repeat on the opposite side. You can now use the portion of the belt that crosses the door's edge as a handle.

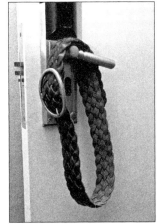
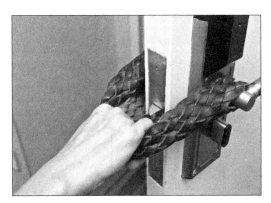

Grab the belt, palm down, with your right hand.

Place your feet on either side of the door, pressing the door between them. Your feet should be directly below the doorknobs, so that you're straddling the door. Be sure that you have good traction with the floor.

Lean back until your right arm is fully extended, with your left arm at your side. Bend your knees about 45 degrees while keeping your back straight, in a neutral posture.

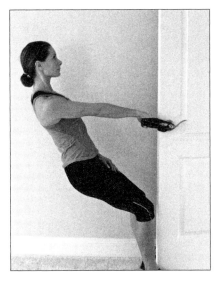
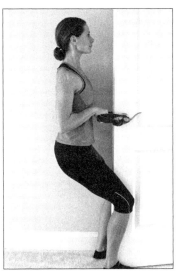

Keeping your knees bent and your feet flat on the ground, pull your upper torso all the way to the hand of your working arm. Both your shoulder blades should remain retracted.

Return to the starting position in a controlled motion, stretching your right arm until it is fully extended once again.

Need to take it down a notch? Move your feet back slightly.

WATCH the workout—
SCAN here

6. One-arm Let Me Ins with knees slightly bent and 2-second pauses

Once your supporting hand is touching your upper torso, hold the position for 2 seconds. Keep your midsection tight and both shoulder blades squeezed together.

7. One-arm Let Me Ins

This exercise is just like one-arm Let Me Ins with knees slightly bent, except your knees will remain bent at 90 degrees with your thighs parallel to the ground.

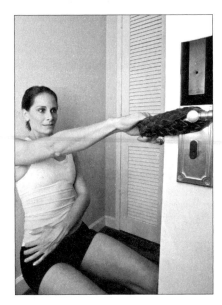 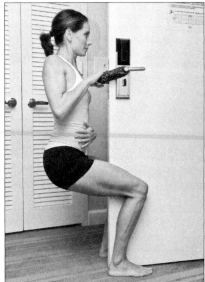

Need to take it down a notch? Straighten your legs slightly.

8. One-arm Let Me Ins with 2-second pauses

Once your supporting hand is touching your upper torso, hold that position for 2 seconds. Keep your midsection tight and keep both shoulder blades squeezed together.

9. Let Me Ups with knees bent 90 degrees

Lie on your back underneath anything that is stable enough for you to pull yourself up, such as a desk, table, or some type of pole supported by two surfaces (more on this later). It should be just beyond arm's reach above you (about waist height if you are standing). It's okay if the surface is a bit closer than arm's length, but it's not ideal, because it will restrict your movement a little.

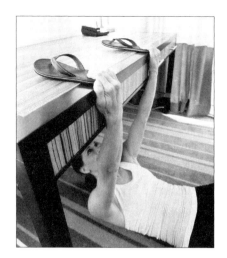

Lie under the thing that you are going to use to pull yourself up, so that the lower portion of your chest is directly below where your hands will be.

Reach up and grab the bar or surface, with your hands slightly wider than shoulder width apart if possible.

Bend your knees, and bring your feet toward your butt; keep your feet flat on the ground.

Raise your butt off the ground so your body is in a rigid line from your knees to your shoulders.

Pull your chest up to the surface or bar. Only your feet should be touching the ground.

Slowly lower yourself all the way back down without letting go of the surface, always keeping your butt off the ground and your body in a rigid line from your knees to your shoulders.

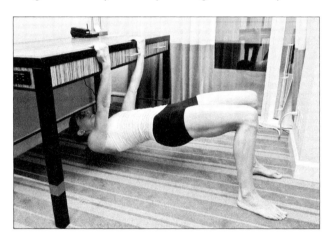 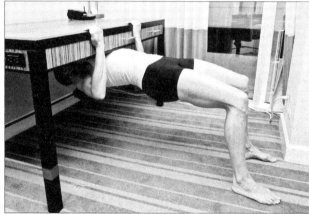

If the surface that you're grabbing onto is slick, try placing something with grip, such as flip-flops, under your hands.

It can make it easier on your hands if you drape a towel or any cloth over the surface, just at the edge where you grip. Then squeeze the towel(s) to the desk between your thumb and fingers as you do this exercise.

Need to take it down a notch? Tuck your feet under your butt. In this position, only the balls of your feet will be touching the ground. Use your legs to assist in the movement by engaging the quadriceps (the front of the thighs) as if doing leg extensions.

Finding something to do Let Me Ups on:

   Look around your home and be creative. I first started doing these by laying a sturdy broom across the tops of two tall stereo speakers. You can also use a mop or any pole that won't break. You only need to lay it across two even surfaces about waist height above the floor: chairs, tables, file cabinets, you name it. Unless you have a very strong pole, place the two even surfaces just barely wider than shoulder width apart. Be sure the pole is steady and will not slide one way or the other. (If your surfaces are wooden, you can put two small nails around the broomstick on each surface to hold it in place, then, if you want, remove the nails when you're done and put them aside for the next time.)

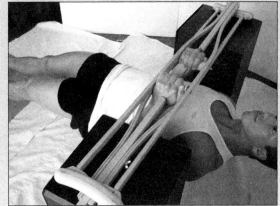

   Got an old pair of crutches? Lay them across the two surfaces facing opposite ways so that the handles are about a foot apart and above your chest and get to work! Crutches are absolutely ideal tools for this exercise.

   Keep in mind that you don't need any kind of pole. You can use a table or desk as well. This is what I do while on the road training in a hotel room, which is the majority of the time. You can also buy one of my handy Bodyweight Bars, which allow you to do this and every other exercise in the book without the use of anything else.

10. Let Me Ups with knees bent 90 degrees and 1-second pauses

Hold the lower portion of your sternum (the bony area between the bottom of your chest and top of your abdomen) against the supporting surface for 1 second.

11. Let Me Ups with knees bent 90 degrees and 2-second pauses

Hold the lower portion of your sternum against the supporting surface for 2 seconds.

12. Let Me Ups with knees slightly bent

Lie on your back underneath anything that is stable enough for you to pull yourself up, such as a sturdy desk, table, or bar.

Reach up and grab the surface or bar, with your hands slightly wider than shoulder width apart.

Bend your knees 45 degrees, with your heels on the ground.

Raise your butt off the ground so your body is in a rigid line, from your knees to your shoulders.

Pull your lower chest up to the surface or bar.

Only your heels should be touching the ground.

Slowly lower yourself back down without letting go of the surface.

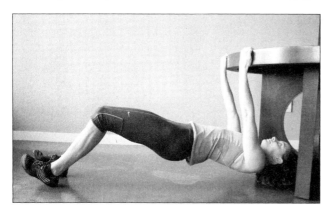 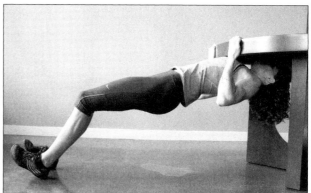

Need to take it down a notch?
Move your feet a little closer to your butt.

13. Let Me Ups with knees slightly bent and 1-second pauses

Hold the lower portion of your sternum against the supporting surface for 1 second.

14. Let Me Ups with knees slightly bent and 2-second pauses

Hold the lower portion of your sternum against the supporting surface for 2 seconds.

15. Let Me Ups with legs straight

Lie on your back underneath anything that is stable enough for you to pull yourself up, such as a sturdy desk, table, or bar.

Lie so that your chest is directly under the surface or bar.

Reach up and grab the surface or bar, with your hands slightly wider than shoulder width apart. Your legs should be straight.

Keeping your body in a straight line, from your heels to your shoulders, pull your lower chest up to the surface or bar. Only your heels should be touching the ground.

Slowly lower yourself back down without letting go of the surface.

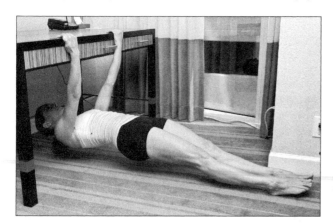 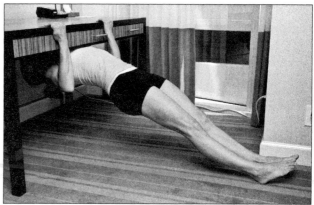

You may have to reposition yourself after the first rep so that the bottom of your chest touches between your hands at the top of the movement. This makes the exercise much easier.

Need to take it down a notch? Bend your knees slightly.

16. Let Me Ups with legs straight and 1-second pauses

Hold the lower portion of your sternum against the supporting surface for 1 second.

17. Let Me Ups with legs straight and 2-second pauses

Hold the lower portion of your sternum against the supporting surface for 2 seconds.

18. Let Me Ups with feet elevated

Lie on your back underneath anything that is stable enough for you to pull yourself up, such as a sturdy desk, table, or bar.

Lie so that your chest is directly under the surface or bar.

You'll also need a chair or something about knee height on which to place your feet.

Reach up and grab the surface or bar, with your hands slightly wider than shoulder width apart.

While holding on to the surface, elevate your feet onto a knee-height surface, making a straight line from your heels to your shoulders.

Keeping your body in a straight line, from your heels to your shoulders, pull your lower chest up to the surface or bar.

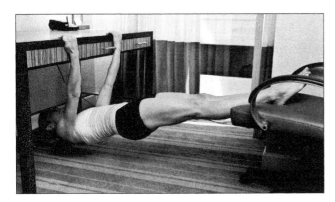 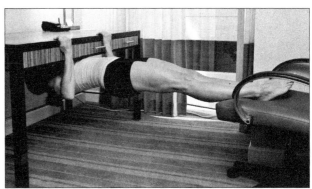

Slowly lower yourself back down without letting go of the surface.

You may have to reposition yourself after the first rep so that the bottom of your chest touches between your hands at the top of the movement.

Need to take it down a notch? Use a slightly lower than knee-height surface.

19. Assisted Pull-ups

Anywhere you can find a sturdy door, you can do Pull-ups.

Wedge a doorstop or towel either underneath the door or over one of the hinges to keep it from swinging.

Open the door halfway and fold a towel, T-shirt, or cloth over the top. Give yourself just enough padding to make your hands comfortable.

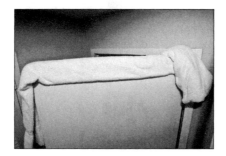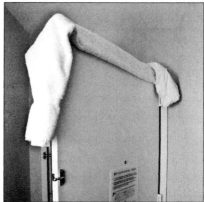

Use a surface, such as a chair, to put your feet on, so you can use your legs to assist yourself throughout the movement. Be sure that your chin comes over the top of the door when you are standing up on the surface. Shorter women might need a higher surface such as a sturdy table or stepladder. Or they can stack something like phone books or a crate on a chair, so long as it is secure.

Facing the door, place your hands slightly wider than shoulder width apart on the cloth over the door.

Standing on your raised surface, bend your knees until your arms are at full extension.

Using your legs to assist *as little as possible*, pull yourself up against the door until your chin is over the top.

Lower yourself slowly until your elbows are straight.

The upward portion of the movement should take about 3 seconds, as should the downward part.

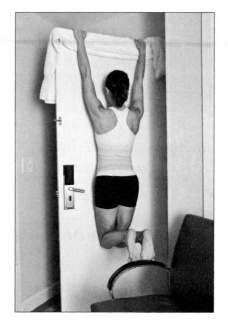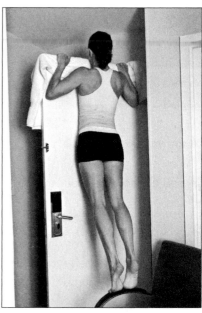

You'll be able to do this variation for all reps the first time you try it, because of the assistance from your legs. Move on to the next Pulling exercise only after you feel comfortable with this variation.

20. Assisted Pull-ups with 2-second unassisted negative

If you can do so safely, once your chin is over the supporting surface, lift your feet into the air and lower yourself to the bottom position without the assistance of your legs. The descent should take 2 seconds. Use your legs as needed on the way up.

Need to take it down a notch? If you get to the point where you can't control your descent, finish the set by assisting yourself on the way up and on the way down.

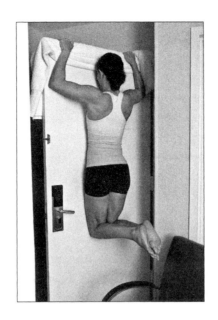

21. Assisted Pull-ups with 3-second unassisted negative

Use your legs as little as possible to help you up. Then lift your feet up and slowly lower yourself from the top position to the fully extended position. The descent should take 3 seconds.

Need to take it down a notch? If you get to the point where you can't control your descent, finish the set by assisting yourself on the way up and on the way down.

22. Assisted Pull-ups with 4-second unassisted negative

Use your legs as little as possible to help you up. Then lift your feet up and slowly lower yourself from the top position to the fully extended position. The descent should take 4 seconds.

Need to take it down a notch? If you get to the point where you can't control your descent, finish the set by assisting yourself on the way up and on the way down.

23. Assisted Pull-ups with 3-second unassisted negative and 1-second pauses

Without the assistance of your legs, pause for 1 second once your chin is over the supporting surface. Your feet should be raised up in the air. Next, with your feet still raised, slowly lower yourself from the top position to the fully extended position. The descent should take 3 seconds.

Need to take it down a notch? If you get to the point where you can't control your descent, finish the set by assisting yourself on the way up and on the way down.

24. Assisted Pull-ups with 4-second unassisted negative and 1-second pauses

Without the assistance of your legs, hold your chin over the supporting surface for 1 second. The descent should take 4 seconds.

25. Pull-ups

Perform this exercise without the assistance of your legs and without pauses. Make sure that your chin clears the top and your arms are fully extended at the bottom.

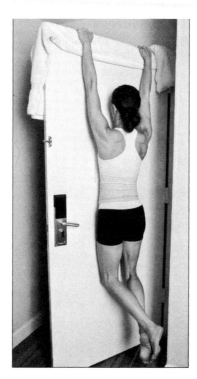 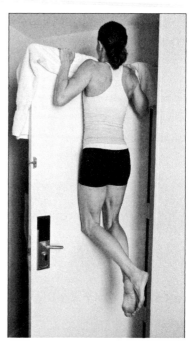

Need to take it down a notch? If you get to the point where you can't do any more unassisted Pull-ups, finish the set by assisting yourself on the way up and getting an unassisted descent.

Ready to kick it up a notch? Once you've conquered this exercise for all prescribed reps, you can continue to progress by adding pauses and/or 1 rep to each set. For example: 3 x 8 would become 3 x 9, and so on. You can also go to YouAreYourOwnGym.com for more-advanced progressions.

Squatting Exercises

Squatting movements work your glutes, quads, hamstrings, lower back, core, and calves.

Top Tips

Focus on keeping your knees steady. Your knees should always point in the same direction as your toes. Novice trainees often make the mistake of allowing their knees to buckle in toward each other.

Your knees should not protrude forward of your toes. Always sink your hips down and back as if sitting onto a chair.

As much as possible, maintain a slight inverse arch in your back with your shoulder blades squeezed together, your chin slightly retracted, and your chest out.

It's okay and necessary to lean forward, especially with single-limb movements.

SQUATTING EXERCISES IN ORDER OF DIFFICULTY:

1. Therapy Sumo Squats
2. Therapy Sumo Squats with 2-second pauses
3. Therapy Squats
4. Therapy Squats with 2-second pauses
5. Overhead Squats
6. Overhead Squats with 2-second pauses
7. Side Lunges
8. Side Lunges with 1-second pauses
9. Side Lunges with 2-second pauses
10. Bulgarian Split Squats with arms overhead
11. Bulgarian Split Squats with arms overhead and 1-second pauses
12. Bulgarian Split Squats with arms overhead and 2-second pauses
13. One-legged Squats off knee-height surface
14. Assisted One-legged Squats
15. Assisted One-legged Squats with 1-second pauses
16. Assisted One-legged Squats with 2-second pauses
17. Assisted Pistols
18. Assisted Pistols with 1-second pauses
19. Assisted Pistols with 2-second pauses
20. One-legged Squats
21. One-legged Squats with 1-second pauses
22. One-legged Squats with 2-second pauses
23. Pistols
24. Pistols with 1-second pauses
25. Pistols with 2-second pauses

1. Therapy Sumo Squats

Face a wall with your feet a little wider than shoulder width apart and toes pointing outward at 45 degrees. Your toes should be about one foot's length from the wall.

Gently place your fingers on the back of your head.

Sink your hips back and down, as if sitting onto a chair behind you, while keeping a slight arch in your back and your feet flat on the ground.

Throughout the movement, be sure your knees are pointing in the same direction as your toes.

Once the tops of your thighs are parallel to the ground, reverse the motion until you are standing erect in the starting position again. The wall helps you perfect your Squatting form, by ensuring that you sit back and maintain an adequate arch in your back.

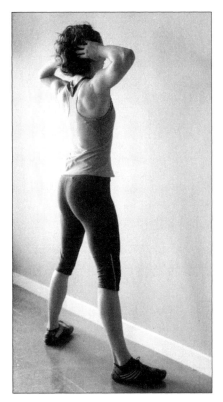 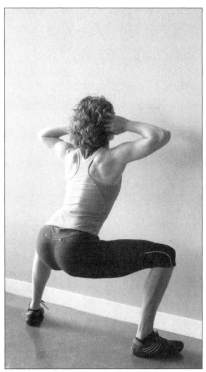

Need to take it down a notch? Reverse the motion before the tops of your thighs are parallel to the ground. Increase your range of motion as you get stronger and/or your flexibility increases.

2. Therapy Sumo Squats with 2-second pauses

Hold the bottom of the Squat for 2 seconds, when the tops of your thighs are parallel to the ground.

WATCH the workout—
SCAN here

3. Therapy Squats

This movement is the same as the Therapy Sumo Squat, except your feet will be no wider than shoulder width apart, with your toes pointing outward no more than 20 degrees. The motion can be reversed when the bottoms of your thighs are parallel to the ground.

Need to take it down a notch? Reverse the motion before the bottoms of your thighs are at or below parallel to the ground. Increase your range of motion as you get stronger and/or your flexibility increases.

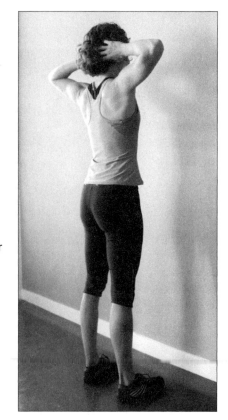
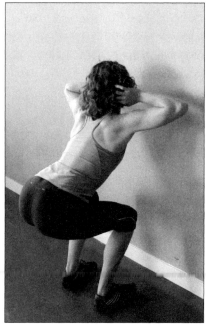

4. Therapy Squats with 2-second pauses

Hold the bottom of the Squat for 2 seconds, when the bottoms of your thighs are at or below parallel to the ground.

5. Overhead Squats

Perform a Squat while holding a light object, such as a towel, overhead, with your elbows locked straight out and your hands slightly wider than shoulder width apart. The top of your thighs should be parallel to the ground before reversing the motion.

For added stability, shrug your shoulders as high as possible throughout the movement, lock your elbows, and act as if you were trying to pull the object apart.

Your feet should be slightly wider than shoulder width apart, with your toes pointing outward about 20 degrees. Your feet should remain flat on the ground, and your knees should point in the same direction as your toes.

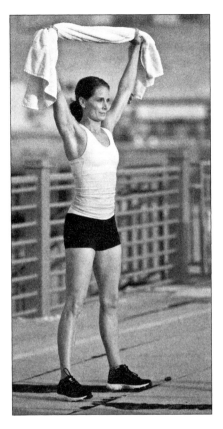
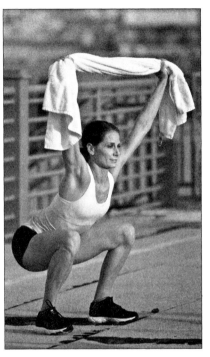

Need to take it down a notch? Reverse the motion before the tops of your thighs are parallel to the ground. Increase your range of motion as you get stronger and/or your flexibility increases.

WATCH the workout—
SCAN here

6. Overhead Squats with 2-second pauses

Hold the bottom of the Squat for 2 seconds, when the tops of your thighs are parallel to the ground.

HOOYA!

Most guys don't have the shoulder flexibility to balance an object above their center of gravity, which causes the object to fall forward while they are in the bottom position. This can make for a great gender challenge that you're very likely to win. Next time a guy starts running his mouth about how strong he is, start with just a bar or another light object and add 5 pounds at a time until he buckles before you—the champion.

7. Side Lunges

Stand upright with your feet together and your hands stretched out straight in front of you, Frankenstein style.

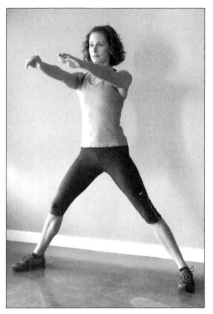
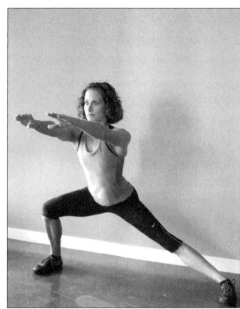

Take a wide step to the side with your right foot, your toes pointing straight ahead. As your right foot comes in contact with the ground, shift your weight onto it.

Keeping your shoulder blades back and an inverse arch in your back, lower your hips down and back as if sitting onto a chair. Your left leg should stay straight.

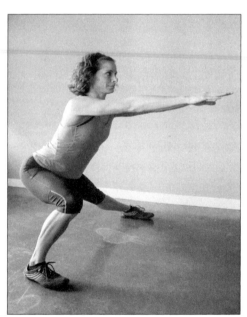

Come down until the bottom of your right thigh is at or below parallel to the ground.

Return to the starting position by forcefully pushing off your right heel.

After performing all reps on the right side, switch legs and repeat the same number of reps on your left side.

Need to take it down a notch? Reverse the lunge before your working leg is parallel to the ground. Increase the range of motion as you get stronger.

8. Side Lunges with 1-second pauses

Hold the bottom position of the movement, with the bottom of your working thigh at or below parallel to the ground, for 1 second.

9. Side Lunges with 2-second pauses

Hold the bottom position of the movement, with the bottom of your working thigh at or below parallel to the ground, for 2 seconds.

10. Bulgarian Split Squats with arms overhead

Stand facing away from a knee-height surface, such as a chair or bed, and take one slightly longer than normal step forward, away from the surface. You can also use the third step on a staircase.

Place the top of your left foot on the knee-height surface behind you, and raise your arms straight overhead.

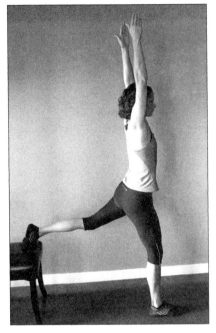
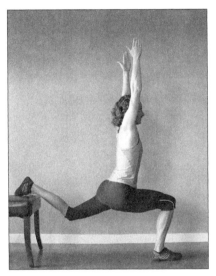

For comfort, you can put a pillow on the surface, and place your foot on the pillow, if you like.

Throughout the movement, keep your arms straight overhead. Sink your hips back and down, until at least the bottom of your right thigh is parallel to the ground. If the knee of your right leg is going forward past your toes, you need to sit back more.

Reverse the motion until your right leg is straight again.

Repeat the same number of reps using your left leg.

This is a great exercise that develops strength, balance, and flexibility, preparing you for more-difficult one-legged exercises.

Need to take it down a notch? Don't hold your arms overhead if you're having balance issues. Once your balance improves, begin to hold your arms overhead. You can also use a slightly smaller range of motion, then increase it as your balance and strength improve.

11. Bulgarian Split Squats with arms overhead and 1-second pauses

Hold the bottom position, with the bottom of your working thigh at or below parallel to the ground, for 1 second.

12. Bulgarian Split Squats with arms overhead and 2-second pauses

Hold the bottom position, with the bottom of your working thigh at or below parallel to the ground, for 2 seconds.

13. One-legged Squats off knee-height surface

Stand facing away from a knee-height surface that is just behind you, such as a chair or ottoman. The back of your knees should almost touch the surface behind you.

Put your arms straight out, Frankenstein style, and raise your left leg slightly off the ground.

While maintaining a slight arch in your back, gently sit back onto the surface in a controlled motion, without "flopping" onto it.

Reverse the motion by standing up without rocking forward.

The foot of your supporting leg should remain flat on the ground throughout this movement.

As soon as you're finished, perform the same number of reps using the opposite leg.

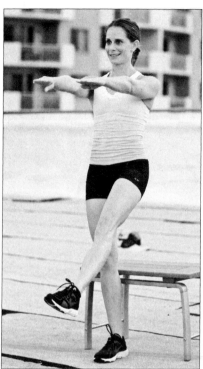 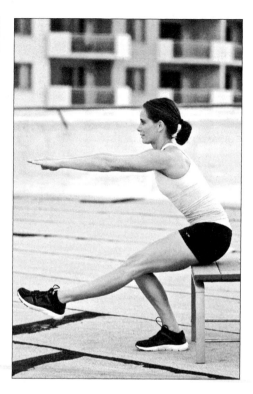

Need to take it down a notch? Use a surface that is slightly higher than knee height. Find progressively lower surfaces to sit on as you get stronger, until you can use a knee-height surface. An easy way to make a surface a little higher, and adjustable, is to add phone books or magazines.

14. Assisted One-legged Squats

A great place to do these is in an open doorway.

Stand one step back from the doorway. Reach forward and grab hold of the opposite sides of the doorway at waist level.

You should be positioned so that you need to bend forward slightly to grab the doorway with extended arms.

Lift one leg off the ground a few inches. Use your straight arms to stabilize and take weight off your working leg as you sit back, without actively pulling unless you have to.

Lower your hips until the

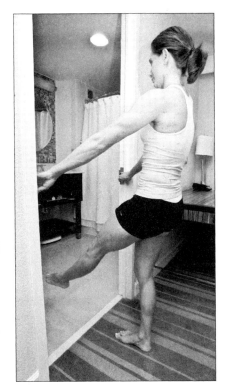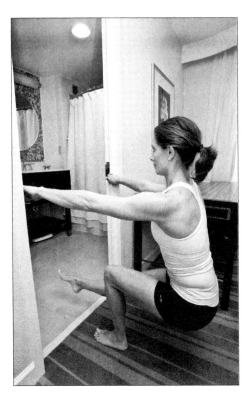

bottom of your supporting thigh is at least parallel to the ground. Reverse the motion and return to the starting position. Keep your arms as straight as possible throughout this movement.

Need to take it down a notch? Bend your elbows and pull yourself up lightly with your arms.

15. Assisted One-legged Squats with 1-second pauses

Hold the bottom position, with the bottom of your working leg at least parallel to the ground, for 1 second.

16. Assisted One-legged Squats with 2-second pauses

Hold the bottom position, with the bottom of your working leg at least parallel to the ground, for 2 seconds.

17. Assisted Pistols

This exercise is the same as the Assisted One-legged Squat, except you won't reverse the motion, by standing up, until the top of your thigh is below parallel to the floor. But don't go so far down that your weight rests on your calf.

Need to take it down a notch?

Bend your elbows and pull lightly with your arms for greater assistance.

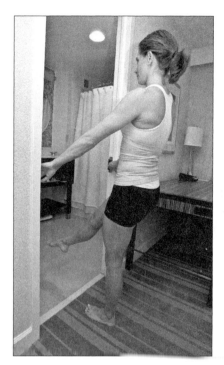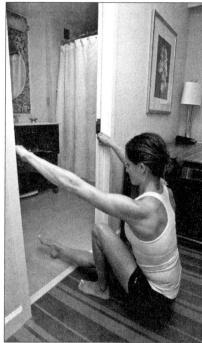

18. Assisted Pistols with 1-second pauses

Hold the bottom position, with the top of your working thigh at or below parallel, for 1 second. Don't allow your weight to rest on your calf.

19. Assisted Pistols with 2-second pauses

Hold the bottom position, with the top of your working thigh at or below parallel, for 2 seconds. Don't allow your weight to rest on your calf.

20. One-legged Squats

Stand upright with your arms raised straight out in front of you.

Lift your left leg slightly off the ground.

Lower your hips back and down, as if sitting onto a chair behind you, while reaching forward with your arms and keeping your left leg off the ground.

Once the bottom of your right thigh is at or below parallel to the ground, reverse the motion and stand back up. The heel of your right leg should remain on the ground.

Switch legs when you are done, and perform the same number of repetitions.

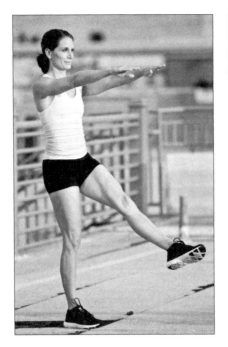
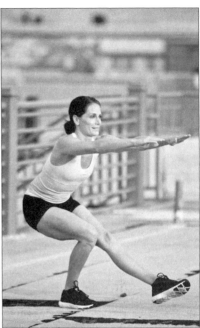

Need to take it down a notch? Reverse the motion before the bottom of your working thigh is parallel to the ground. Then increase your range of motion as you get stronger.

21. One-legged Squats with 1-second pauses

Hold the bottom position, with the bottom of your working leg at least parallel to the ground, for 1 second.

22. One-legged Squats with 2-second pauses

Hold the bottom position, with the bottom of your working leg at least parallel to the ground, for 2 seconds.

23. Pistols

This movement is just like the One-legged Squat except that you will lower your hips until the *top* of your supporting thigh is below parallel to the ground. Don't go so far down that all your weight is resting on your calf in the bottom position.

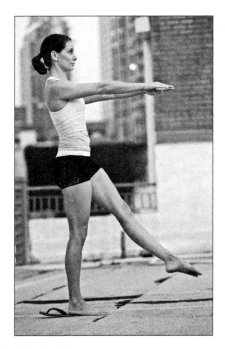

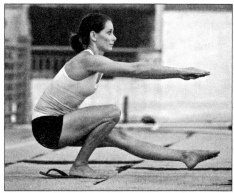

If you have the tendency to fall backward while in the bottom position, try sliding something thin, like a flip-flop, under your working heel. Slowly wean yourself from using this crutch by placing progressively thinner objects under your heel as your ankle flexibility improves.

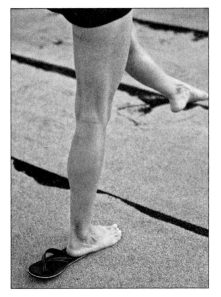

Need to take it down a notch? Gently sit onto a mid-shin-height surface, such as a stepping stool, suitcase, or stair, and stand up off it. Try not to use momentum, by rocking forward, to stand up.

HOOYA!

Hey, if you've made it this far—outstanding! The pistol is the mother of all leg exercises. It creates the perfect balance of strength, stability, and flexibility. As for athletic ability, you're now in the top one percent of all people. Please come by YouAreYourOwnGym.com to share your success with me and with others.

24. Pistols with 1-second pauses

Hold the bottom position, with the top of your working leg below parallel to the ground, for 1 second. Don't rest on your calf in the bottom position.

25. Pistols with 2-second pauses

Hold the bottom position, with the top of your working leg below parallel to the ground, for 2 seconds. Again, don't rest on your calf in the bottom position.

Ready to kick it up a notch? Once you've mastered this variation, you can continue to progress by adding repetitions to each set. You can also start trying this exercise with your arms extended overhead or while holding water jugs or a weighted backpack in your hands. Go to YouAreYourOwnGym.com for more-advanced progressions.

In-line Pushing Exercises

These movements start with your arms in line with your body, so that a straight line is formed from your wrists to your hips. These exercises focus on your shoulders, triceps, and core.

Top Tips

The starting positions for these exercises are all identical, with the only variable being the elevation of your hands or feet.

Be sure to maintain a slight inverse arch in your back, chest and butt out, throughout these movements. This will help elongate your spine and stretch your hamstrings and calves in the starting positions.

An imaginary line drawn between your wrists, shoulders, and hips should always be straight, so that the emphasis remains on your shoulders rather than your chest muscles. Avoid shrugging your shoulders toward your ears during these movements. Instead, keep your shoulders pulled down and back, into your body.

After each rep, take a brief moment to check your posture: straight line from wrists to hips, slight arch in back, and straight legs.

IN-LINE PUSHING EXERCISES IN ORDER OF DIFFICULTY:

1. Military Presses with hands elevated hip height
2. Military Presses with hands elevated hip height and 1-second pauses
3. Military Presses with hands elevated hip height and 2-second pauses
4. Military Presses with hands elevated knee height
5. Military Presses with hands elevated knee height and 1-second pauses
6. Military Presses with hands elevated knee height and 2-second pauses
7. Half Dive-bombers with hands elevated knee height
8. Half Dive-bombers with hands elevated knee height and 1-second pauses
9. Half Dive-bombers with hands elevated knee height and 2-second pauses
10. Military Presses
11. Military Presses with 1-second pauses
12. Military Presses with 2-second pauses
13. Military Presses with feet elevated knee height
14. Military Presses with feet elevated knee height and 1-second pauses
15. Military Presses with feet elevated knee height and 2-second pauses
16. Dive-bombers without reversal
17. Dive-bombers without reversal with 1-second pauses
18. Dive-bombers without reversal with 2-second pauses
19. Half Dive-bombers
20. Half Dive-bombers with 1-second pauses
21. Half Dive-bombers with 2-second pauses
22. Dive-bombers
23. Dive-bombers with 1-second pauses on the way down
24. Dive-bombers with 2-second pauses on the way down
25. Dive-bombers with 1-second pauses on the way up

1. Military Presses with hands elevated hip height

Find a sturdy surface at approximately hip height, such as a countertop, staircase, table, or desk. Step back from the surface and place your hands as if you are about to do a Push-up on it. You can also place your hands against a wall at hip height.

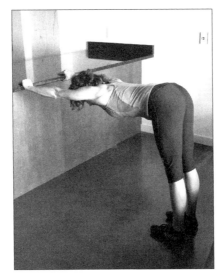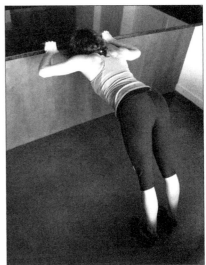

Your hands should be slightly wider than shoulder width apart.

With your arms straight, bring your hips back until a straight line is formed from your wrists to your hips. Your feet should be only slightly behind your hips. Your upper body should be parallel to the floor with a slight arch in your lower back.

If you don't have the hamstring flexibility to maintain a slight arch in your lower back, just keep it as straight as possible.

While keeping your chest down and a slight arch in your lower back, bend at the elbows until the top of your head almost touches the supporting surface between your hands.

Reverse the motion until your arms are at full extension, while keeping your chest down and butt poked up.

Need to take it down a notch? Having your feet slightly closer to the surface makes this exercise easier. As you progress, inch your feet back until your feet are slightly behind your hips.

WATCH the workout—
SCAN here

2. Military Presses with hands elevated hip height and 1-second pauses

Once your head is almost touching the supporting surface, hold for a 1-second count.

3. Military Presses with hands elevated hip height and 2-second pauses

Once your head is almost touching the supporting surface, hold for a 2-second count.

4. Military Presses with hands elevated knee height

Find a sturdy object at approximately knee height—such as a chair, staircase, ottoman, or coffee table—on which to place your hands. If you need to, move the object against a wall to keep it from sliding.

From the starting position of a Push-up, bring your hips back until a straight line is formed from your wrists to your hips. While keeping your legs straight, bend your elbows, lowering your head until it almost touches the supporting surface between you hands. Reverse the motion, while keeping your chest down, until your arms are fully extended again.

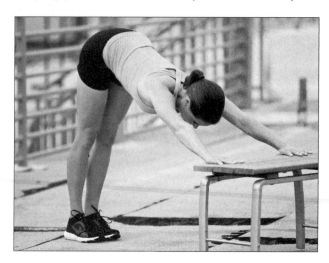 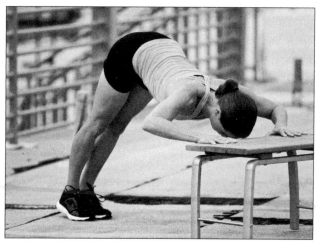

Need to take it down a notch?
A slightly more than knee-height surface will make this exercise easier.

5. Military Presses with hands elevated knee height and 1-second pauses

Hold for a 1-second count once your head is almost touching the supporting surface.

6. Military Presses with hands elevated knee height and 2-second pauses

Hold for a 2-second count once your head is almost touching the supporting surface.

7. Half Dive-bombers with hands elevated knee height

Find a sturdy knee-height surface, such as a chair, ottoman, or coffee table. If you're using an object that might slide, back it against a wall before beginning.

Step back from the object. With your elbows straight, place your hands on it as if getting into a Push-up position. Both your feet and hands should be slightly wider than shoulder width apart.

While keeping your arms extended, bring your hips back until a straight line is formed from your wrists to your hips. Your body should form a right angle. Throughout the movement, keep your legs and back as straight as possible.

While keeping your chest down, bend at the elbows until your head almost touches the supporting surface.

Continue to bend at the elbows, bringing your head forward, until your upper chest swoops down between your hands.

Reverse the motion, extending your elbows, while again keeping your chest down.

Need to take it down a notch?

Using a supporting surface that is slightly higher than knee height makes the exercise easier.

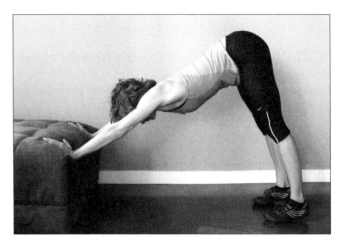

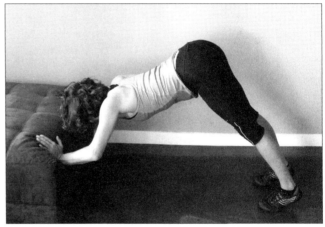

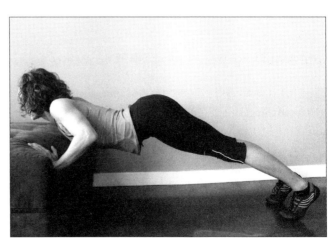

WATCH the workout—
SCAN here

8. Half Dive-bombers with hands elevated knee height and 1-second pauses

Hold for a 1-second count once your upper chest is between your hands.

9. Half Dive-bombers with hands elevated knee height and 2-second pauses

Hold for a 2-second count once your upper chest is between your hands.

10. Military Presses

Position yourself on the floor in the classic Push-up position. Both your feet and hands should be slightly wider than shoulder width apart.

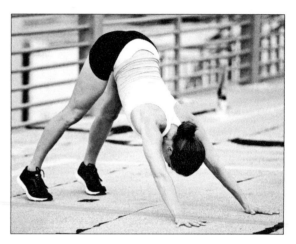

With your arms straight, bring your hips back and up until a straight line is formed from your wrists to your hips. Your body should form a right angle at the hips, and you should have a slight arch in your back. If you don't have the hamstring flexibility to maintain an arch in this position, just keep your lower back as straight as possible.

While keeping your torso in line with your arms and a slight arch in your lower back, bend at the elbows until the top of your head almost touches the ground between your hands.

Reverse the motion until your arms are at full extension.

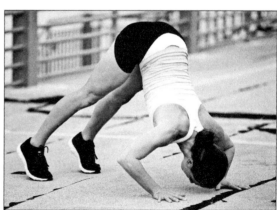

Need to take it down a notch? Use a shorter range of motion, slowly increasing it as you get stronger.

11. Military Presses with 1-second pauses

Hold for a 1-second count once your head is almost touching the ground.

12. Military Presses with 2-second pauses

Hold for a 2-second count once your head is almost touching the ground.

13. Military Presses with feet elevated knee height

Place your feet on a knee-height surface, such as a chair or staircase, and place your hands on the ground so that you are in a Push-up position. Then continue as with a standard military press.

Need to take it down a notch? Elevate your feet on a slightly lower than knee-height surface.

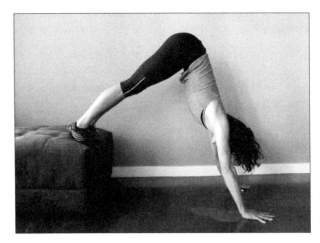

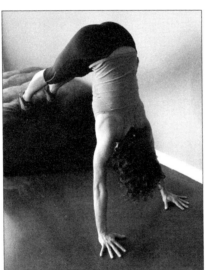
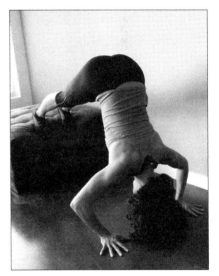

14. Military Presses with feet elevated knee height and 1-second pauses

Hold for a 1-second count once your head is almost touching the ground.

15. Military Presses with feet elevated knee height and 2-second pauses

Hold for a 2-second count once your head is almost touching the ground.

16. Dive-bombers without reversal

Get in the starting position for a Push-up.

   Both your feet and hands should be slightly wider than shoulder width apart. With your arms straight, bring your hips up and back until a straight line is formed from your wrists to your hips.

   Sticking your chest out, swoop your upper body down in an arc so that your chest almost brushes the floor (at which point you should be in the bottom position of a classic Push-up, except with your butt poked out a bit). Then sweep your head and shoulders up as high as possible, until your back is fully arched and you're staring straight ahead, with your pelvis only about an inch off the ground. This should be one fluid motion.

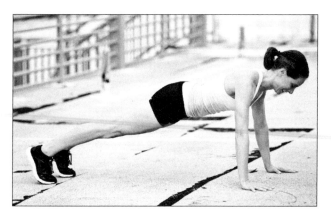
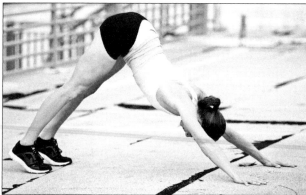
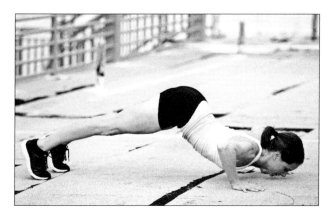
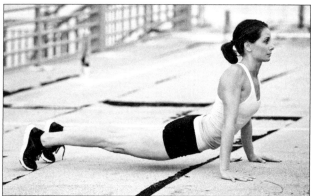

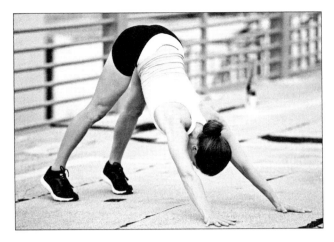

From this position, lift your butt up and back until you are in the starting position again. Tighten your core to help your body contract on the way up.

Need to take it down a notch? Spreading your legs wider makes this exercise a bit easier.

17. Dive-bombers without reversal with 1-second pauses

Pause for a 1-second count once you're looking straight ahead with your pelvis barely off the ground.

18. Dive-bombers without reversal with 2-second pauses

Pause for a 2-second count once you're looking straight ahead with your pelvis barely off the ground.

19. Half Dive-bombers

Get in the starting position for a Push-up, with your hands and feet on the ground. Both your feet and hands should be slightly wider than shoulder width apart. With your arms straight, bring your hips up and back until a straight line is formed from your wrists to your hips.

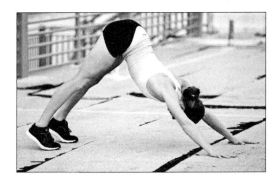

Lower your body, bending at your elbows until your head almost touches the ground between your hands, as in a military press.

But here's the difference: Continue to dive down, lifting your head, until your upper chest is just above the ground and between your hands.

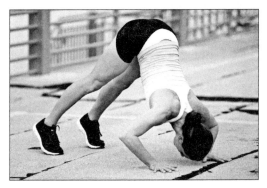

Reverse the motion, keeping your torso and arms in line. While pushing to extend your arms back to the starting position, keep your midsection tight and contracted.

Using your midsection to bring your torso and legs toward each other takes some of the stress off your shoulders and arms.

Need to take it down a notch? You can reverse the movement before your upper chest is between your hands to shorten the range of motion and make the exercise a bit easier. Increase the range of motion as you get stronger.

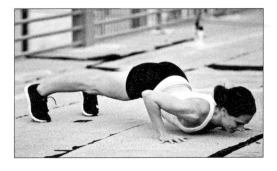

20. Half Dive-bombers with 1-second pauses

Once your upper chest is between your hands, hold it there for a 1-second count.

21. Half Dive-bombers with 2-second pauses

Once your upper chest is between your hands, hold it there for a 2-second count.

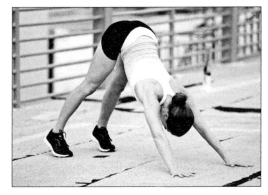

22. Dive-bombers

Get in the starting position for a Push-up, with your hands and feet on the ground. Both your feet and hands should be slightly wider than shoulder width apart. With your arms straight, bring your hips up and back until a straight line is formed from your wrists to your hips.

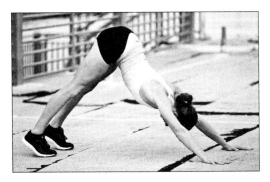

Sticking out your chest, swoop your upper body down in an arc so that your chest almost brushes the floor (at which point you should be in the bottom position of a Push-up, except with your butt poked out). Then sweep your head and shoulders up as high as possible, until your back is fully arched and you're staring straight ahead, with your pelvis only slightly off the ground.

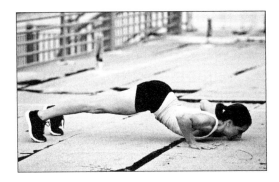

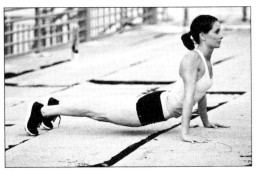

Reverse the motion, again sweeping your chest close to the ground (so that you are again in the bottom

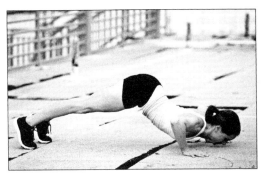

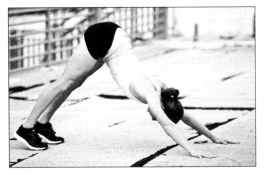

position of a classic Push-up but with your butt poking up), and only then push your body back—this is the hardest part!—until your arms are straight and in line with your back and your butt's up in the air again. On the way up to the starting position, focus on keeping your back arched and your core actively engaged. This will take some of the workload off your shoulders and arms.

Need to take it down a notch? Spread your legs wider than shoulder width apart.

23. Dive-bombers with 1-second pauses on the way down

On the way down, once your chest is between your hands, pause for 1 second.

24. Dive-bombers with 2-second pauses on the way down

On the way down, once your chest is between your hands, pause for 2 seconds.

25. Dive-bombers with 1-second pauses on the way up

On the way back to the starting position, once your chest is between your hands, pause for 1 second before pushing your butt back into the air.

Ready to kick it up a notch? Add 1 rep to each set. Once you can do all sets with the additional rep, add another, and so on. You can also go to YouAreYourOwnGym.com for more-advanced progressions.

HOOYA!

Once you can do this exercise, you're officially in the elite club! This is one heck of an exercise that is sure to keep you lean, strong, and limber. Don't be surprised if people start asking you for training sessions. Find me on YouAreYourOwnGym.com to share your success (and to send me my 50 percent cut!).

Perpendicular Pushing Exercises

These are movements that start with your arms perpendicular to your body. This emphasizes your chest, triceps, shoulders, and core, especially your abdominals.

Top Tips

Throughout these movements, flex your abdominals, keeping your pelvis tilted forward, and retract your chin slightly, to maintain a straight line from head to heels.

Be certain not to let your pelvis drop toward the ground or let your butt stick up in the air at all. Weak form means a weak core. Keep your midsection tight!

Always position your hands so that the lower part of your sternum is between your palms in the bottom position.

Keep your shoulders pulled down and back into your body, rather than shrugged toward your ears while pushing.

PERPENDICULAR PUSHING EXERCISES IN ORDER OF DIFFICULTY:

1. Push-ups with hands elevated sternum height
2. Push-ups with hands elevated sternum height and 2-second pauses
3. Push-ups with hands elevated hip height
4. Push-ups with hands elevated hip height and 2-second pauses
5. Close-grip Push-ups with hands elevated hip height
6. Close-grip Push-ups with hands elevated hip height and 1-second pauses
7. Close-grip Push-ups with hands elevated hip height and 2-second pauses
8. Push-ups with hands elevated knee height
9. Push-ups with hands elevated knee height and 1-second pauses
10. Push-ups with hands elevated knee height and 2-second pauses
11. Close-grip Push-ups with hands elevated knee height
12. Close-grip Push-ups with hands elevated knee height and 1-second pauses
13. Close-grip Push-ups with hands elevated knee height and 2-second pauses
14. Push-ups
15. Push-ups with 1-second pauses
16. Push-ups with 2-second pauses
17. Close-grip Push-ups
18. Close-grip Push-ups with 1-second pauses
19. Close-grip Push-ups with 2-second pauses
20. Push-ups with feet elevated knee height
21. Push-ups with feet elevated knee height and 1-second pauses
22. Push-ups with feet elevated knee height and 2-second pauses
23. One-arm Push-ups with hand elevated hip height
24. One-arm Push-ups with hand elevated hip height and 1-second pauses
25. One-arm Push-ups with hand elevated hip height and 2-second pauses

1. Push-ups with hands elevated sternum height

Stand one big step back from a wall. With your feet together, place your hands on the wall at sternum height (the bony area between the bottom of your chest and top of your abdomen). Your hands should be placed slightly wider than shoulder width apart, and you should be leaning forward slightly.

While keeping a straight line from head to heels, bend your elbows until your nose almost touches the wall. The bottom of your chest should be between your hands.

Push off the wall until your arms are fully extended to complete the repetition.

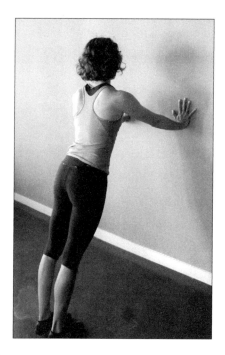 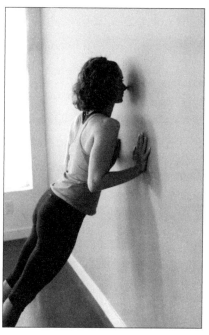

Need to take it down a notch? Stand slightly closer to the wall.

WATCH the workout—
SCAN here

2. Push-ups with hands elevated sternum height and 2-second pauses

With your nose almost touching the wall, hold for a 2-second count.

3. Push-ups with hands elevated hip height

With your feet together, place your hands slightly wider than shoulder width apart, on a sturdy hip-height surface such as a countertop, table, or desk.

While keeping a straight line from head to heels, lower your body, bending at your elbows, until the bottom of your chest almost touches between your hands.

Push yourself back up until your arms are fully extended.

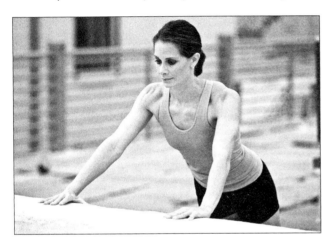 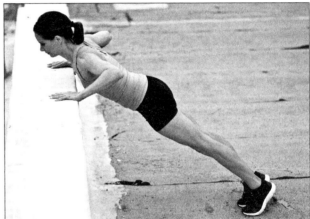

Need to take it down a notch?
Use a slightly higher than hip-height surface.

4. Push-ups with hands elevated hip height and 2-second pauses

Hold the bottom position, with your chest almost touching the supporting surface, for a 2-second count.

5. Close-grip Push-ups with hands elevated hip height

These are like Push-ups with hands elevated hip height, except your hands will be close enough that your thumbs can touch. Reverse the movement just before your chest touches your hands.

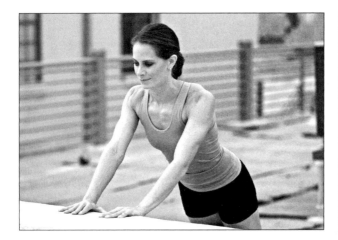 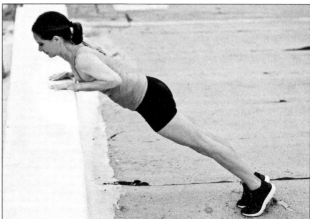

Need to take it down a notch? Use a slightly higher than hip-height surface.

6. Close-grip Push-ups with hands elevated hip height and 1-second pauses

Hold the bottom position, with your chest almost touching your hands, for a 1-second count.

7. Close-grip Push-ups with hands elevated hip height and 2-second pauses

Hold the bottom position, with your chest almost touching your hands, for a 2-second count.

WATCH the workout—
SCAN here

8. Push-ups with hands elevated knee height

With your feet together, place your hands slightly wider than shoulder width apart on a knee-height surface, such as a chair, ottoman, or coffee table.

While keeping a straight line from head to heels, lower your body, bending at your elbows, until the bottom of your chest almost touches between your hands. Push off until your arms are fully extended to complete the repetition.

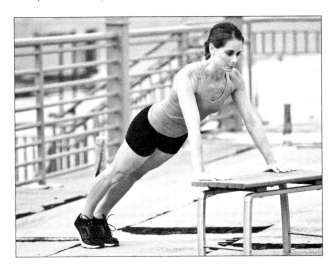 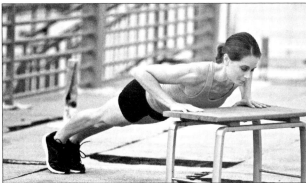

Need to take it down a notch? Use a slightly higher than knee-height surface.

9. Push-ups with hands elevated knee height and 1-second pauses

Hold the bottom position, with your chest almost touching the supporting surface, for 1 second.

10. Push-ups with hands elevated knee height and 2-second pauses

Hold the bottom position, with your chest almost touching the supporting surface, for 2 seconds.

11. Close-grip Push-ups with hands elevated knee height

These are like Push-ups with hands elevated knee height, except your hands will be close enough that your thumbs can touch. Reverse the movement just before your chest touches your hands.

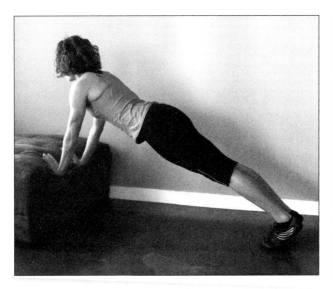 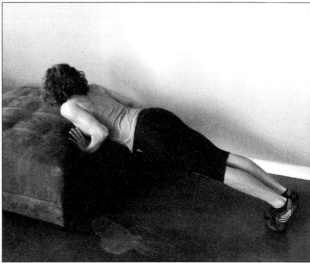

Need to take it down a notch?
Use a slightly higher than knee-height surface.

12. Close-grip Push-ups with hands elevated knee height and 1-second pauses

Hold the bottom position, with your chest almost touching your hands, for a 1-second count.

13. Close-grip Push-ups with hands elevated knee height and 2-second pauses

Hold the bottom position, with your chest almost touching your hands, for a 2-second count.

14. Push-ups

Kneel down on the floor, lean forward, and place your hands slightly wider than shoulder width apart on the ground.

Lift your knees off the ground so that you are straight from head to heels, with only your hands and feet touching the ground. Throughout the entire movement, your body should remain absolutely straight.

Lower your chest until it almost touches the ground. Reverse the motion, pushing yourself back up, until you're in the starting position with your arms fully extended.

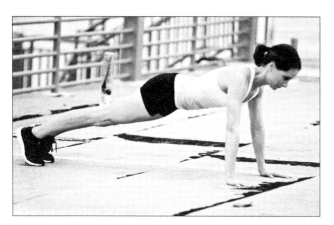 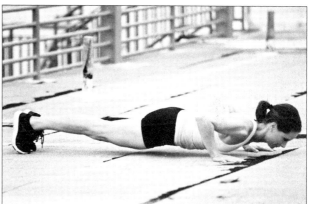

Need to take it down a notch? Spread your legs.

15. Push-ups with 1-second pauses

Hold the bottom position, with your chest almost touching the floor, for a 1-second count.

16. Push-ups with 2-second pauses

Hold the bottom position, with your chest almost touching the floor, for a 2-second count.

17. Close-grip Push-ups

This one is like the Push-up except your hands will be close enough for your thumbs to touch.

Reverse the movement just before your chest touches your hands.

Need to take it down a notch? Spread your legs.

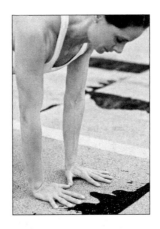

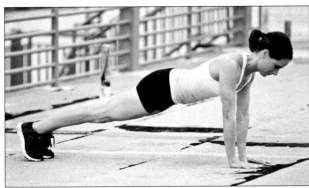
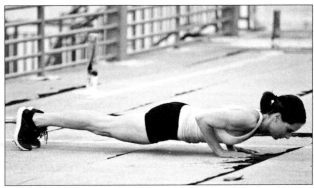

18. Close-grip Push-ups with 1-second pauses

Hold the bottom position, with your chest almost touching your hands, for a 1-second count.

19. Close-grip Push-ups with 2-second pauses

Hold the bottom position, with your chest almost touching your hands, for a 2-second count.

20. Push-ups with feet elevated knee height

Get in a Push-up position with your hands on the ground and feet elevated on a knee-height surface. Throughout the entire movement, your body should be in a straight line. From your heels to your neck, nothing should be bent.

Let yourself descend in a controlled fall until your nose almost touches the ground.

Reverse the motion, and return to the starting position.

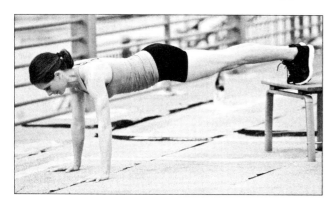 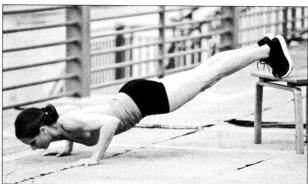

Need to take it down a notch? Use a slightly lower than knee-height surface.

21. Push-ups with feet elevated knee height and 1-second pauses

Hold the bottom position, with your nose almost touching the floor, for a 1-second count.

22. Push-ups with feet elevated knee height and 2-second pauses

Hold the bottom position, with your nose almost touching the floor, for a 2-second count.

23. One-arm Push-ups with hand elevated hip height

Lean over and place your hands on a hip-height surface, such as a desk or countertop, just as you would for a Close-grip Push-up.

Put your right hand behind your back. Place your right leg out to the right, using it like a kickstand. A straight line should be maintained from your left heel to your left shoulder.

Always keeping your shoulders parallel to the surface, come down as far as possible before pushing yourself back up.

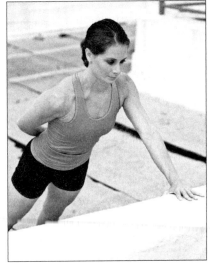

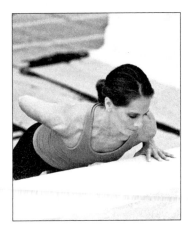

Keep the elbow of your working arm tucked in to your ribs. And pay special attention to keeping your shoulders squared and down away from your neck. You should remain on your toes throughout the movement.

You should really feel your abs working to keep your body straight!

Need to take it down a notch? Elevate your hands on a slightly higher than hip-height surface.

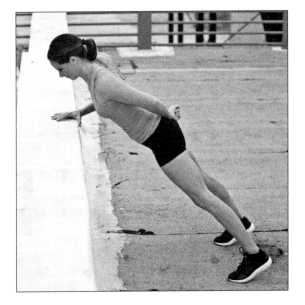

HOOYA!

If you're advanced enough to do this exercise with good form, you're quite simply awesome! And you'll soon discover that this is the greatest of all "ab" exercises. It is one of the few movements that develops rotational strength, because of the torque it applies to your midsection.

24. One-arm Push-ups with hand elevated hip height and 1-second pauses

With your chest almost touching the supporting surface, hold for a 1-second count before pushing yourself back up.

25. One-arm Push-ups with hand elevated hip height and 2-second pauses

With your chest almost touching the supporting surface, hold for a 2-second count before pushing yourself back up.

Ready to kick it up a notch?
Place your hands onto progressively lower surfaces. When you make it to the floor, you'll be in better shape than G.I. Jane, because by following my instructions you'll have much better form than Demi Moore did in that movie.

HOOYA!

Go to YouAreYourOwnGym.com for even more advanced progressions. If you've made it this far, help motivate others by leaving a short success story.

Bending Exercises

These are exercises that mainly involve bending at the waist. Bending movements work your legs, glutes, back, core, and often shoulders and triceps too.

Top Tips
For all the Bending exercises, maintain a slight inverse arch in your back, so that your chest and butt stick out slightly.

Keep your chin slightly retracted and your shoulders pulled down and back, rather than shrugged toward your ears.

BENDING EXERCISES IN ORDER OF DIFFICULTY:

1. Good Mornings
2. Good Mornings with 1-second pauses
3. Good Mornings with 2-second pauses
4. Warriors
5. Warriors with 1-second pauses
6. Warriors with 2-second pauses
7. Hip Extensions
8. Hip Extensions with 1-second pauses
9. Hip Extensions with 2-second pauses
10. Hip Raisers
11. Hip Raisers with 1-second pauses
12. Hip Raisers with 2-second pauses
13. One-legged Hip Extensions
14. One-legged Hip Extensions with 1-second pauses
15. One-legged Hip Extensions with 2-second pauses
16. One-legged Hip Raisers
17. One-legged Hip Raisers with 1-second pauses
18. One-legged Hip Raisers with 2-second pauses
19. One-legged Romanian Dead Lifts
20. One-legged Romanian Dead Lifts with 1-second pauses
21. One-legged Romanian Dead Lifts with 2-second pauses
22. One-legged Warriors
23. One-legged Warriors with 1-second pauses
24. One-legged Warriors with 2-second pauses
25. One-legged Warriors Holding Object Overhead

1. Good Mornings

Stand with your feet hip width apart and your fingertips gently touching behind your head.

Bend forward, only at the hip, keeping an inverse arch in your back (chest and butt out). You should feel tension in the backs of your legs (hamstrings) and lower back. Bend over until going any farther requires rounding your lower back.

Reverse the motion while maintaining the arch in your back. You should bend only at the hips.

Need to take it down a notch? Let your arms hang down in front of you, or place your hands on your hips.

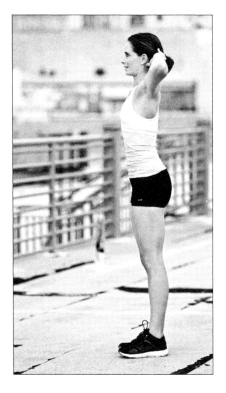 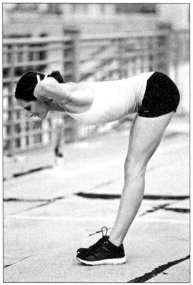

2. Good Mornings with 1-second pauses

Hold the bottom of the movement for 1 second once you feel tightness in your hamstrings.

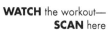

WATCH the workout—
SCAN here

3. Good Mornings with 2-second pauses

Hold for 2 seconds once you feel tightness in your hamstrings.

4. Warriors

This exercise is just like Good Mornings, except your arms are held straight overhead. Your palms should be turned in toward each other, with your upper arms right next to your ears throughout the movement.

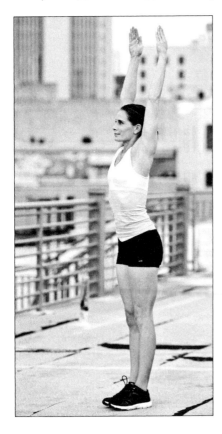

Need to take it down a notch? Bend the elbows.

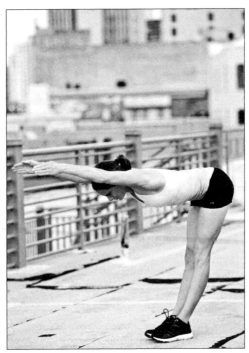

5. Warriors with 1-second pauses

Hold the bottom of the movement for 1 second once you feel tightness in your hamstrings.

6. Warriors with 2-second pauses

Hold for 2 seconds once you feel tightness in your hamstrings.

7. Hip Extensions

Lie flat on your back with your arms at your sides and your heels resting on a knee-height surface, such as a chair. Your knees should be bent at a 90-degree angle.

Now, using only your legs, push your hips upward as high as you can or until your thighs and upper torso form a slight outward arch.

Slowly lower your hips back to the starting position.

Keep your knees and feet together throughout the movement.

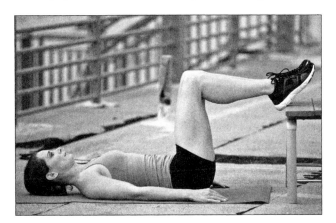 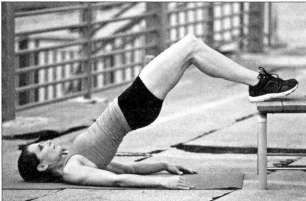

Need to take it down a notch? To make this exercise easier, you can decrease the range of motion by not pushing your hips all the way up.

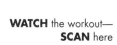 **WATCH** the workout—
SCAN here

8. Hip Extensions with 1-second pauses

Hold the top position for 1 second, really squeezing with your glutes and hamstrings.

9. Hip Extensions with 2-second pauses

Hold the top position for 2 seconds, really squeezing with your glutes and hamstrings.

10. Hip Raisers

Sit on the ground with your back straight up and your legs straight out.

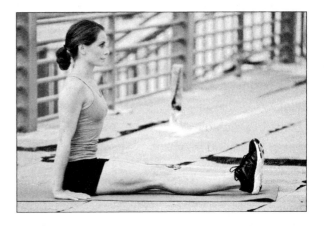

Put your arms to your sides, with your palms flat on the ground on either side of your butt and your fingers pointing in the direction of your feet or just slightly outward.

Throughout the exercise, act as if trying to rotate your hands outward, without actually rotating your hands. This will help to retract your shoulder blades.

Keep your arms nearly straight, without locking out your elbows. Raise your pelvis upward so that the soles of your feet now are flat on the floor and your knees are bent at a 90-degree angle above your feet. Your body—from your shoulders down through your hips and upper thighs, all the way to your knees—should be in a straight line. Let your head fall backward so that you are looking upward.

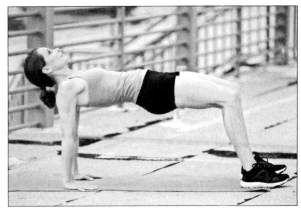

Lower yourself all the way back to the starting position before beginning the next rep.

Need to take it down a notch? Don't return all the way to the starting position. Instead, keep your legs bent at a 90-degree angle and reverse the motion as soon as your butt touches the ground.

11. Hip Raisers with 1-second pauses

Add a 1-second hold to the top of the movement, really squeezing your glutes and hamstrings.

12. Hip Raisers with 2-second pauses

Add a 2-second hold to the top of the movement, really squeezing your glutes and hamstrings.

13. One-legged Hip Extensions

Lie flat on your back with your arms at your side, the heel of your right leg resting on a knee-height surface such as a chair, and your left leg pointing straight up in the air. Your right leg should be bent at about a 90-degree angle.

Now, using only your right leg, push your hips upward as high as you can. A slight outward arch should be formed from your left knee to your shoulders.

Then slowly lower your hips back to the starting position.

Need to take it down a notch? Don't go all the way up. Then increase your range of motion as your strength and flexibility improve.

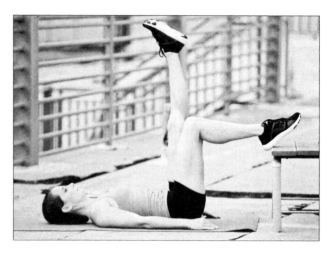

14. One-legged Hip Extensions with 1-second pauses

Add a 1-second hold to the top of the movement, really squeezing your glutes and hamstrings.

15. One-legged Hip Extensions with 2-second pauses

Add a 2-second hold to the top of the movement, again really squeezing your glutes and hamstrings.

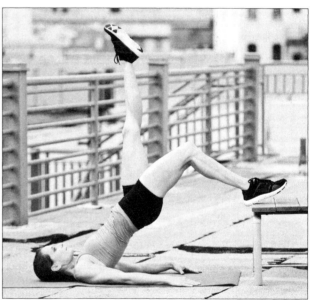

16. One-legged Hip Raisers

Sit on the ground with your back straight up and your legs straight out. Put your arms to your sides, with your palms flat on the ground on either side of your butt and your fingers pointing in the direction of your feet or slightly outward. Throughout the exercise, act as if trying to rotate your hands outward. This will help to retract your shoulder blades.

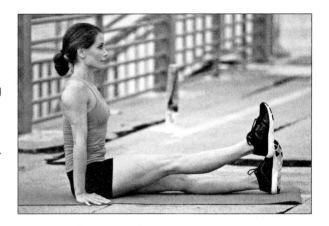

Raise your right leg a couple of inches off the ground.

Keep your arms nearly straight, without locking out your elbows. Using only your left leg, raise your pelvis upward until your left foot is flat on the floor. Your body—from your shoulders down through the left thigh—should be in a straight line or have a slight upward arch. Let your head fall backward so that you are looking upward. Your right leg should point up at a 45-degree angle or more throughout the exercise.

Lower yourself all the way back to the starting position before beginning the next rep.

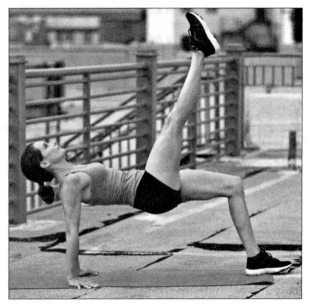

Need to take it down a notch? Don't return all the way to the starting position. Instead, keep your working leg bent at a 90-degree angle and reverse the motion when your butt touches the floor.

17. One-legged Hip Raisers with 1-second pauses

Add a 1-second hold to the top of the movement, really squeezing your glutes and hamstrings.

18. One-legged Hip Raisers with 2-second pauses

Add a 2-second hold to the top of the movement, again really squeezing your glutes and hamstrings.

19. One-legged Romanian Dead Lifts

Stand upright, with your left leg raised slightly behind you and the toes of your right foot pointing straight ahead.

Keep a slight arch in your back, your shoulders perfectly level, and reach down with both arms while raising your left leg straight behind you as you lower your upper body.

Your knees should remain only very slightly bent throughout the motion, and your elevated

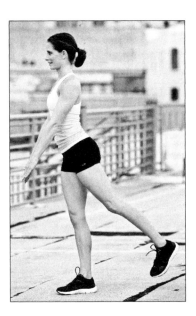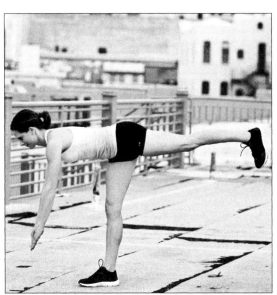

leg should remain in a straight line with your upper torso. The goal here is to form a line from your left heel to your head.

It's helpful to focus on leading with the elevated leg. Let your upper torso follow as you pick up your leg. Try to keep the toes of your elevated leg from pointing outward.

Once your upper body and elevated leg are at or slightly below parallel to the ground—so that your body is basically forming a T—reverse the motion and return to the upright position.

You can use a shorter range of motion if you don't have the flexibility to get parallel to the ground. But be sure to go as far as you can with each rep while still maintaining a slight inverse arch in your back.

Need to take it down a notch?
Set your elevated leg down for stability between reps.

20. One-legged Romanian Dead Lifts with 1-second pauses

Hold for 1 second in the bottom position once you feel a stretch in your supporting leg's hamstrings.

21. One-legged Romanian Dead Lifts with 2-second pauses

Hold for 2 seconds once you feel a stretch in your supporting leg's hamstrings.

22. One-legged Warriors

This exercise is just like a One-legged Romanian Dead Lift, except your arms are extended straight overhead. The palms of your hands should be facing each other, with your upper arms remaining right next to your ears. Keep your shoulders pulled in to your body rather than shrugged to your ears.

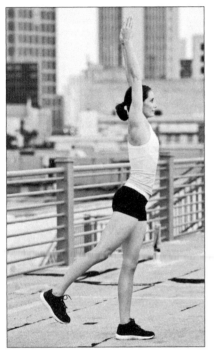

Need to take it down a notch? Set your elevated leg down for stability between reps.

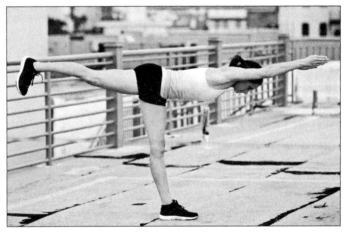

23. One-legged Warriors with 1-second pauses

Hold for 1 second once you feel a stretch in your supporting leg's hamstrings.

24. One-legged Warriors with 2-second pauses

Hold for 2 seconds once you feel a stretch in your supporting leg's hamstrings.

25. One-legged Warriors Holding Object Overhead

Stand upright, with your right leg slightly elevated behind you and your arms straight overhead, holding a 3-to-5-pound object, such as a phone book, backpack, or large water bottle. Your palms should be turned toward each other.

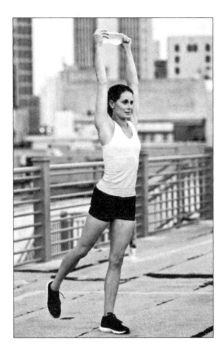
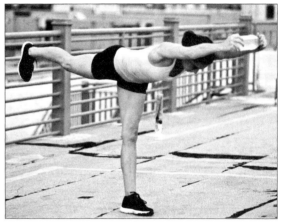

Keeping a slight arch in your back and your shoulders level, bend forward while raising your right leg straight behind you. Your knees should remain only slightly bent, and your elevated leg should remain in a straight line with the upper torso.

It's helpful to lead with your rear leg. Focus on picking up your back leg rather than leaning forward. The key here is to keep a basically straight line between your hands and your raised heel.

Once your upper body and elevated leg are parallel to the ground, forming a T, reverse the motion and return to the upright position.

Need to take it down a notch? Find a lighter object.

Ready to kick it up a notch? Once you've conquered this exercise, you can continue to increase its difficulty by holding gradually heavier objects and incorporating pauses. It doesn't take a lot of weight to make this exercise much harder. I recommend stepping it up in only 1-to-3-pound increments. Use a backpack, and add light objects as you get stronger. You can also add reps to each set. Go to YouAreYourOwnGym.com for even more advanced progressions.

HOOYA!

This is a phenomenal exercise that develops strength, flexibility, and balance. If you're doing this movement with an object overhead, you have the posterior development of a goddess, the stability of an oak, and the ability to tackle nearly anything in this world.

PART III

Body by You
Nutrition

7

The Basics

Anyone who has tried to eat healthfully can attest to the huge profits reaped, such as improved energy, mood, and body composition. Proper nutrition is absolutely essential, no matter your goals.

It is incredibly easy to eat healthy. Rather than providing complex charts, or listing foods that leave you scratching your head about how to actually put them together, or offering meal plans that are difficult to follow unless you have a private chef, I'm going to show you how to understand food so you can always rely on your own knowledge about what to eat. I'll give you some sample meals to get you started, but I want to educate, not control your every move. In the end, you need to read your groceries, not some chapter in a book.

In a Nutshell

Here are the four simple keys to looking and feeling your best with proper nutrition:

1. Whenever possible, each different food you eat in a meal should have only one ingredient, with the exception of some seasoning if you want it.
2. In each meal, maintain a fairly even ratio of calories coming from fat, carbs, and protein.

3. Eat roughly every three hours. That's five small meals a day.
4. Go to YouAreYourOwnGym.com, click on "Nutrition," and find out how many calories you should consume in each meal, depending on your goal: fat loss (and how much), toning, or putting on a little weight.

That's it.

No, really, that is it.

But to succeed, unless you're already a nutrition junkie, you're going to need the why and how to easily implement this program. So please read on. . . .

Expanding Your Knowledge, Not Your Waistline

For millions of years, our ancestors survived purely on seven food types: vegetables, fruits, nuts, seeds, meats, eggs, and fish. Typically the women gathered the nuts, seeds, fruits, and vegetables, while the men hunted for meat. Together, these food sources provided the necessary components of a complete diet that sustained healthy living. Climate, geography, and luck mainly determined how balanced these sources were. But, remember, regardless of how much of each food our ancestors ate, these were the *only* foods available to them. Naturally, our bodies have adapted to their consumption.

It wasn't until about ten thousand years ago, with the cultivation of plants and the domestication of animals, that large quantities of breads, potatoes, rice, pasta, and dairy became available. These relatively new sources of calories were the main reason our complex societies were able to develop, and our overpopulation is to a large degree due to them.

However, for millions of years our bodies evolved on diets without any of these. The relatively minuscule time span since the domestication of plants and animals has not prepared us to live healthy lives with diets consisting of too many breads, pastas, rice, and potatoes. Yes, life expectancy has greatly increased in this time span, but that can be attributed not to new foods but rather to man's no longer having to live on the go while dealing with hunger, thirst, illness, injuries, extreme cold, and dangerous animals.

So think of these new calories as little more than fillers. If you find yourself overwhelmed by nutritional definitions and rules, just ask yourself this: For millions of years before the domestication of plants and animals, what did people eat?

To better understand the "why" behind this simple philosophy and how to tailor it to your needs, we have to first understand some basic terms of nutrition.

Macronutrients

Macronutrients consist of proteins, fats, and carbohydrates. Contrary to common belief, each is a *necessary* part of a healthy and effective nutritional plan, regardless of your goals; excluding any one of them (the way some popular diets would have you do) will cause you to feel unsatisfied and tired.

Micronutrients

Micronutrients, such as vitamins and minerals, are required in minuscule amounts to maintain optimal health. The importance of these micronutrients is often overlooked, despite the fact that imbalances of them cause poor performance, illness, and even death.

Today's diets in Western civilization, while usually calorie-rich, are often deficient in micronutrients, because many of those calories don't come from natural sources.

Since I realize that it's not always possible to eat perfectly, I suggest taking a greens supplement such as Green Vibrance, a powder made up of organically grown and very nutrient-dense vegetation such as alfalfa sprouts, carrots, zucchini, broccoli sprouts, green beans, and spinach.

Calories

Food is an energy source, and calories are a measurement of how much energy is in our food. Calorie selection and quantity are important to improving body composition and performance.

Fats

Fats are calorie-rich, with nine calories per gram versus four calories for protein and carbs, but that doesn't make them bad. It is important to understand that dietary fat does not automatically convert to body fat and that fats in the correct proportions are extremely important to optimal health. Fats improve the taste of food, aid in longer-lasting fullness, slow the absorption of carbs, provide a good energy source, improve brain function, regulate hormones, reduce inflammation, reduce chances of cancer, and even reduce chances of heart disease when eaten in appropriate proportion.

Low-fat diets leave people tired and constantly craving more food. The satiety that you'll get from a little extra fat in your diet will allow you to comfortably eat fewer calories than you would without the fats.

HOOYA!

Trimming the Fat with . . . Fat

Maybe you're thinking, "How can this be right? I cut fats out of my diet once and lost weight!"

True, but you didn't lose weight because you cut fat out of your diet; you lost weight because you were consuming fewer total calories. Just as much weight would have been lost with an equivalent calorie intake that had an even split between the three macronutrients: protein, carbs, and fats.

With the fat, you would have lost the same weight with fewer cravings and been much more likely to keep it off. Low-fat diets are miserable and unsustainable. Contrary to common practice, it is easier to sustain a calorie deficit with a bit of fat in each meal. Dietary fats do not automatically convert to body fat, but excess calories do.

Saturated and Unsaturated

There are two types of dietary fat: saturated and unsaturated. Saturated fats are derived mainly from animal sources and foods containing hydrogenated oil. Unsaturated fats come from plant sources such as nuts, seeds, avocados, olive oil, flaxseed oil, and fish.

About one-third of your calories should come from fats, mainly unsaturated. Regularly eating a small palmful of trail mix, half an avocado, a tablespoon of flaxseed oil in your protein shake, olive oil on your salad, and plenty of fish will provide you with the unsaturated fats that you need. The saturated fats will take care of themselves, as they are a part of the meats, eggs, and dairy we eat for protein. Saturated fats should not come from foods such as french fries, butter, potato chips, or other junk foods.

Protein

Protein breaks down into amino acids, which are the building blocks used to repair and regenerate all cells, including your muscles. Adequate protein intake is essential to maintain and grow muscle. Protein makes you feel full faster than fats or carbs, which is beneficial if you're on a tight diet. It's got four calories per gram, and major sources include poultry, meat, fish, dairy products, soy products, and eggs.

Daily, we should aim to consume an even split of protein, carbs, and fats.

It might be tough at first, but when your mind is craving something loaded with carbs, try eating some protein instead. Believe me, your "hunger" will disappear.

Carbohydrates (Carbs)

Each gram of carbohydrate contains four calories. All carbohydrates are made of sugar molecules. Carbs are a key source of energy, and they include fruits, vegetables, pastas, breads, cereals, rice, and sweeteners such as table sugar and honey. Paramount in your calorie selection is getting the right kind of carbohydrates.

The Glycemic Index

All carbs must be converted to glucose, a type of sugar, before they are absorbed into the bloodstream. A carb's rate of absorption into the bloodstream, to a large degree, determines its value.

A carb's rate of absorption produces a proportionally strong release of the hormone insulin, which regulates the amount of sugar in the blood. When we consume foods with fast-absorbing sugars, such as soda or fruit juice, a strong insulin reaction depletes blood sugar and converts these carbs to fat, leaving us feeling tired and craving more food to restore normal blood-sugar levels. Consumption of rapidly absorbing carbs is a leading cause of obesity.

To aid us in carb selection, we use a glycemic index. The glycemic index measures the rate of absorption of carbs. A carb that has a low glycemic index absorbs slowly (good), and a carb with a high glycemic index absorbs rapidly (bad). For a comprehensive list of foods and their glycemic indices, go to the "Nutrition" link at YouAreYourOwnGym.com.

You will find that almost all raw vegetables and fruits with higher amounts of fiber, like apples and pears, have a much lower glycemic index than most grain products, which includes everything from breads to pasta to rice. These natural unprocessed sources should be chosen because they have slow rates of absorption, low calorie content, and large amounts of fiber, water, and micronutrients.

The problem with most processed foods that come nicely packaged in pretty boxes is that the sugars from these sources absorb into the bloodstream quickly and provide large amounts of calories with little nutritional value. Especially if you want to lose body fat, your carbs should consist mainly of raw vegetables and whole pieces of fruit with low glycemic indices.

In general, whether eating vegetables, fruits, or other sources of carbs, stick with foods that have a glycemic value of *less* than 55, unless you're looking to gain fat. The occasional higher-glycemic-value foods that we do end up eating (for sanity reasons) should be consumed—within your caloric limits—as part of a meal, with balanced macronutrients and at least some raw vegetables and/or whole pieces of fruit.

HOOYA!

Post-Workout Meal

After your workout, you have a small window of time—about forty-five minutes—when your muscles are especially receptive to nutrients needed for recovery. Because you've caused micro-damage to your muscle fibers and depleted their sugar stores, they hunger for protein and carbs.

This is the one time you want carbs with a high glycemic index. They will quickly resupply the muscles via the rapid insulin reaction that they cause. A protein shake with maltodextrin is an excellent choice. You'll find that most meal supplements with both protein and carbs use maltodextrin for the carb source.

This is also the one time that you do not want to add fat to your shake or meal, since fat will slow the absorption of carbs and therefore blunt the insulin reaction, slowing the rate at which the muscles are resupplied with the nutrients to begin repair and growth.

You're the mission coordinator. Don't miss this critical forty-five-minute window of opportunity to shuttle needed nutrients to your hardworking muscles.

You should be aware that rigorous training of any sort is likely to stimulate your appetite, which, if unchecked, can lead to poor eating. A protein shake is the answer, because it will quickly satiate you and help you build a leaner, stronger body.

Water

Water is the single most important nutrient that we consume. Your brain consists of 90 percent water; blood is 83 percent water, muscle is 75 percent water, and even your bones are 22 percent water. Water is critical to every system of your body. Just some of the benefits of being properly hydrated are aided brain function, kidney function, liver function, detoxification, metabolism, joint lubrication, and nutrient absorption. Some of the downfalls of improper hydration include fatigue, constipation, headaches, dry skin, muscle cramps, irregular blood pressure, and false cravings for food.

Women should drink a minimum of nine cups of water a day. That's 4.5 pints, or about two liters. Beyond that, women's need for water varies depending on size, activity, environment, and overall health. A 155-pound softball player in Miami needs more water than a 90-pound lawyer living in Chicago, for example.

Always stay ahead of your thirst. If you're thirsty, you're already dehydrated. The color of your urine should remain clear or have only a slight yellow tint.

Try to have water near you wherever you go. If you can, it's best to drink filtered tap water. It saves money, and it's the greenest option. We all need to drink water consistently and not just pound water every once in a while to catch up.

HOOYA!

Troubled Waters

The sad reality is that most drinks other than water are crap. There are a few exceptions, like low-fat milk, protein shakes, and herbal teas. If you choose to drink the occasional wine, beer, or cocktail, fine. If you enjoy coffee, okay. But during the rest of your day, day-to-day, try not to drink anything but water.

Sodas that are not diet and most juices are packed with insane amounts of highly glycemic and nutritionally empty calories. An apple is a great source of fiber and vitamins, while apple juice is little more than colored sugar water.

Consider that just one can of non-diet soda typically contains 35 grams of sugar. That's 140 nutritionally useless calories that trigger cravings and fatigue. One soda a day for a year adds up to 51,100 calories, the equivalent of 14.5 pounds of fat! Such fluids promote poor body composition and increase the risk of diabetes and heart disease.

Stick with water. Your body will thank you.

Resting Metabolic Rate (RMR)

Your RMR is the amount of calories needed to sustain all of your body's functions while at rest. A person's RMR accounts for approximately 65 percent of the body's total calorie consumption; activity burns the remainder.

It is governed by several factors. Some are genetically predetermined, while others we can control.

The main factor controlling RMR is lean body mass, which accounts for approximately 80 percent of RMR, and there's only one way to affect lean body mass: Build muscle. RMR decreases by about five percent every decade after thirty, mainly because of the loss of muscle mass associated with aging. Fortunately, our lean body mass can be controlled through proper nutrition and strength training. It takes only a few months of training to recover one or two decades of decrease in RMR. Muscles require calories even while at rest. That is a major reason why effective strength training is so important.

Not only does the muscle gained from strength training boost your metabolism, but the actual workout itself does, too, for up to thirty-six hours after completion. This is one of the main reasons why high-intensity interval training is so much more effective than aerobic activity, which is not intense enough to have a lasting impact.

Frequent meals and strength training are essential for the maintenance and development of muscle. From the lasting metabolic boost of intense workouts and the added muscle gained through those workouts, a much higher resting metabolic rate is achieved.

Overcoming Mindless Eating

Breaking bad eating habits can be hard, especially for those who are very overweight. We need to stop eating like hungry pterodactyls and practice awareness, not only during food selection but also during food consumption.

Too often, instead of eating what we really need, we eat more of the high-calorie processed junk, which just makes us fatter without satisfying the deficiencies that caused the hunger and cravings in the first place.

When we eat healthy and balanced meals, our hunger isn't triggered by unhealthy nutrient deficiencies. Since each meal has protein, fats, and plenty of carbs coming from raw vegetables, our bodies get all the necessary nutrients. It's amazing how few calories satisfy us when our bodies get what they need in each meal. Pay attention to the difference.

Overcoming Emotional Eating

Sometimes, people eat to find temporary satisfaction during emotionally tough situations. But doing so often compounds the problem with regret, lowered self-esteem, weight gain, and potential long-term health effects.

HOOYA!

Don't Forget to Feed the Metabolism

Another way to positively influence metabolism is to provide the body with a steady flow of nutrients. As a survival mechanism during times of starvation, the body adapts by slowing down its metabolism, mainly by cannibalizing calorie-consuming muscle. Frequent meals make the maintenance and development of lean tissue much easier, which in turn makes the shedding of fat easier. Each day you should aim to eat 5 small meals at about 3-hour intervals, and never go hungry.

There is a time to eat, and there is a time to face emotional difficulties. These two should never be mixed. It is a shame to undo months of hard work because of a week's worth of emotional eating. Instead, remain mindful of your meals, and deal with your emotions in another way. Go for a walk, talk to a friend, or work out. Nothing lasts forever. If you absolutely must eat something, chop up a variety of raw vegetables and go to town.

Don't Starve Yourself

Too many people starve themselves to lose weight. That is *never* a good idea. At best, it leads to some short-term loss of water, muscle, and fat. But the strategy will always backfire in the long run.

It's true: To lose fat, you will have to eat fewer calories than you burn. But with a proper diet, you should feel energized and satisfied, not hungry.

Even if you succeed in starving yourself for a long time, this only signals the body to slow down the metabolism and to eat muscle, too, which in the end will pack on the pounds.

The reason why people consume more than they need to begin with is that their diets are not supplying all the needed nutrients. When your body is nutrient-deficient, it signals you to eat. It doesn't matter how many "empty" calories you consume; your body's nutrient deficiencies will trigger ongoing hunger. Starving yourself only compounds these deficiencies. It's inevitable that the cravings eventually win, and, once they do, they grow even stronger. But instead of getting nutrient-rich meals that make up for the deficiencies and allow you to be satisfied with fewer calories, the body just gets more empty calories, which further spurs errant cravings. It's a vicious circle. And while you feel like you're starving yourself, you're actually continuing to get too many unneeded calories. The end result: You feel miserable and there's no benefit.

HOOYA!

Have you heard that eating at night will make you fat? Not true. The calories that you eat at night do not automatically turn to fat. If each day you consume 2,000 calories and you burn 2,000 calories, you will still maintain a caloric balance. It doesn't matter what time of day those calories are consumed.

People who don't eat at night and lose weight do so simply because their caloric intake is reduced, not specifically because they didn't eat at night.

Most of our recovery and repair occurs during REM sleep. Especially when strength-training, having the needed nutrients for this will improve sleep quality and help you lose fat.

The flip side is that it's amazing how satisfying a low-calorie diet can be when all the needed nutrients are provided by mainly natural sources.

Here's the bottom line: One or more decades of neglect can't be undone in a month. If you are very overweight, it may take a year. I know, it seems like forever away. It *will* happen, though—but only if you start now.

Again, this does not mean spending a year on a starvation diet and killing all your free time by working out. It involves only a slight tweak to your life: converting one percent of your time to fast, fun workouts and understanding what you're eating. In fact, you will feel *less* hungry, more satisfied, and more energized. But you will need patience. With it, you will get there. Without it, you cannot. The workouts may be quick, but if you're very overweight, the time it takes to really slim down won't be. That's the reality. Anyone telling you different is lying to you.

8

Read Your Food, Plan Your Food

Nutrition Facts		
Serving Size 1/2 cup dry (40 g)		
Servings Per Container: 13		
Amount Per Serving		
Calories 150	Calories from Fat 25	
		% Daily Value*
Total Fat 3 g		**4%**
Saturated Fat 0.5 g		2%
Trans Fat 0 g		0%
Cholesterol 0 mg		**0%**
Sodium 0 mg		**0%**
Total Carbohydrate 27 g		**9%**
Dietary Fiber 4 g		15%
Sugars 1 g		
Protein 5 g		
Vitamin A		0%
Vitamin C		0%
Calcium		0%
Iron		10%

*Percent Daily Values are based on a 2,000 calorie diet. Your daily values may be higher or lower depending on your calorie needs.

		Calories:	2,000	2,500
Total Fat		Less than	65 g	80 g
Sat. Fat		Less than	20 g	25 g
Cholesterol		Less than	300 mg	300 mg
Sodium		Less than	2,400 mg	2,400 mg
Total Carbohydrate			300 g	375 g
Dietary Fiber			25 g	30 g

When it comes to getting good nutrition, there is perhaps nothing that will serve you better than learning to read and understand food labels. When you do, you can plan your meals with variety and efficiency.

Let me give you an example of how to read your food and fit it into a meal. Here's the nutritional label from regular oatmeal. Optimally, all your food sources should have a single ingredient, as regular oatmeal does. Oatmeal's a great foundation for breakfast—the most crucial, and most commonly neglected, meal.

1. Start at the top and let your eyes drift downward. The first two things to note are "Serving Size" and "Servings Per Container," then, directly under "Amount Per Serving," look at "Calories."

Serving size is as important as the calories. Don't get fooled by some muffin that says it has only 150 calories but 4 servings to the thing. Who buys a muffin and only eats a quarter of it? The calories in an actual helping of that muffin are 600. Ditto with many other junk foods we should avoid. Drinks typically list the calories in one 8-ounce serving, even though no one drinks only 8 ounces as a serving, because a can contains 12 ounces and a bottle 16 to 20 ounces. This is why drink labels are often very misleading, and one true portion usually contains many more calories than an "8-ounce serving."

In this case, with oatmeal, one half-cup serving does make a decent-sized bowl of oatmeal; therefore, the nutritional information does apply to one realistic helping of oatmeal.

2. *Now see where those calories come from.* Your eyes should go down the list to "Total Fat: 3 g."

If, whenever it's practical, we stick to whole foods—foods that have a single ingredient—bad things like trans fat, high cholesterol, and high sodium won't be issues. They should all be very low, as they are with this oatmeal.

Next take a look at "Total Carbohydrates: 27 g."

Four grams of those carbs are "Dietary Fiber." Super, just as most whole foods will be. If these carbs have any sugar at all, it will be minimal and natural.

Last but not least is "Protein: 5 g."

Some vitamins are listed below that, and last is the FDA's basic guide for total macronutrients in sample diets. Frankly, I don't ever look at this, nor do I worry about the percentages of daily values in the right column. Unfortunately, the FDA is still stuck in the Stone Age when it comes to nutrition. Actually, in the Stone Age, people ate better than our government tells us to nowadays.

All this should take about five seconds. Now comes the most important step: placing it into a balanced meal.

3. *Look at the ratio of "Total Fat" to "Total Carbohydrate" to "Protein."*

Each macronutrient should make up about a third of a meal. Remember, it's not about the split of macronutrients in each individual food, it's about the split in the entire meal.

So, in the case of this oatmeal, you have a total fat to total carbohydrate to protein ratio of 3 grams (about 27 calories) to 27 grams (108 calories) to 5 grams (20 calories), and only 150 calories total. You have some room to add a little protein and fat. How much room depends on your goals.

Most women need roughly 2,000 calories each day. If you're just looking to tone up—meaning you want to maintain your overall weight but burn some fat and gain more strength—this is how much you should consume.

If you're looking to add a little weight, consume 2,500 calories a day.

If you're looking to shed the fat, however, you'll want to consume about 1,500 calories a day.

Remember, these are approximations. Again, see the "Nutrition" link on YouAreYourOwnGym.com to calculate exactly how many calories you should consume daily, depending on your goal.

So, if you're looking to drop fat and are consuming 1,500 calories a day, each of your five meals should be about 300 calories. That means 25 grams of protein (100 calories), 25 grams of carbs (100 calories), and about 12 grams of fat (roughly 100 calories).

Back to our oatmeal. Add one medium-sized egg and two egg whites to the meal, and you've got about 300 calories and an even ratio of calories from fat, carbs, and protein. You're good to go. Or even mix protein powder right into the oatmeal, as I often do, and add a quarter of an avocado on the side for the fat. The best way to do this is to mix the protein powder with hot water separately, giving it the consistency of pudding or a little thinner, then stir it into the oatmeal once it's cooked. Might sound yucky, but, done right, it's delicious.

The math is a lot easier than it may sound. And you'll find that within a couple of weeks it becomes second nature.

How to Plan Your Meals

As an example throughout this section, I am going to use a 1,500-calorie diet. Below is an example of what a 1,500-calorie diet could look like. Each meal has a fairly even split of fats, carbs, and protein. The splits don't have to be exact.

With a healthy, even split of macronutrients, you'll be amazed at how satisfying a 300-calorie meal can be. You may even notice that your meals are a bit more than you require. That's fine. Eat until you're satisfied, and no more.

When planning your meals, you'll need to take a look at the nutritional value of the foods that you're planning to eat. Again, for a typical 1,500-calorie shed-the-fat diet, each meal should be about 300 calories, and about 100 calories should come from each macronutrient.

To get an even split of macronutrients in five 300-calorie meals for a 1,500-calorie diet, you'll need about 25 grams of protein, 25 grams of carbs, and 11 grams of fat per meal.

Protein: 25 grams = 100 calories

Carbs: 25 grams = 100 calories

Fat: 11 grams = 99 calories

Total: 299 calories

Remember, the breakdown of these three macronutrients in each meal doesn't need to be exact. Just make sure that every meal has at least some of each, ideally somewhere between 80 and 120 calories. That's 9 to 13 grams of fat and 20 to 30 grams each of carbs and protein per meal.

At first, it is helpful to thoughtfully create 300-calorie meals on paper. Because I recommend eating mainly single-ingredient items, such as fish, meats, eggs, fruits, and veggies, which do not have nutritional labels, I have included a link on my website, at YouAreYourOwnGym.com, that will allow you to easily find the nutritional value of most foods.

SAMPLE MEAL PLAN

Here's an easy-to-prepare 1,500-calorie meal plan. It's not set in stone, just an example of what a good meal plan looks like.

Breakfast—Meal 1

1 banana: 0 grams of fat, 25 grams of carbs, 0 grams of protein

2 medium whole eggs: 11 grams of fat, 0 grams of carbs, 12 grams of protein

3 medium egg whites: 0 grams of fat, 0 grams of carbs, 11 grams of protein

Macronutrient ratio =
11 grams of fat to 25 grams of carbohydrates to 23 grams of protein

(11:25:23)

Fat: 99 calories

Carbs: 100 calories

Protein: 92 calories

Total: 291 calories

or

1 serving of oatmeal: 3 grams of fat, 27 grams of carbs, 5 grams of protein

1 tablespoon of peanut butter: 8 grams of fat, 3 grams of carbs, 4 grams of protein

5 hard-boiled egg whites: 0 grams of fat, 0 grams of carbs, 20 grams of protein

11:30:29

Fat: 99 calories
Carbs: 120 calories
Protein: 116 calories
Total: 335 calories

Mid-Morning—Meal 2

You can make this meal even easier by simply buying a protein powder that already has carbs in it. Just don't forget the fat.

1 scoop of protein powder: 0 grams of fat, 0 grams of carbs, 22 grams of protein

½ cup frozen strawberries: 0 grams of fat, 9 grams of carbs, 0 grams of protein

½ cup apple juice: 0 grams of fat, 15 grams of carbs, 0 grams of protein

1 tablespoon of flaxseed oil: 12 grams of fat, 0 grams of carbs, 0 grams of protein

12:24:22

Fat: 108 calories
Carbs: 96 calories
Protein: 88 calories
Total: 292 calories

Lunch—Meal 3

The next two meals are salads that could be made twice this size and split into two meals for less of a hassle. You would just have to eat the same salad twice in one day. Be sure to mix a variety of different colored vegetables—baby tomatoes, spinach, mushrooms, onions, bell peppers, et cetera. Get creative and try new things. Stay away from the typical and nutritionally lame iceberg lettuce.

1 palm-sized serving of chicken breast: 0 grams of fat, 0 grams of carbs, 27 grams of protein

4 cups mixed vegetables*: 0 grams of fat, 20 grams of carbs, 0 grams of protein

¼ avocado: 9 grams of fat, 4 grams of carbs, 0 grams of protein

1 tablespoon of vinaigrette: 4 grams of fat, 1½ grams of carbs, 0 grams of protein

13:25½:27

Fat: 117 calories
Carbs: 102 calories
Protein: 108 calories
Total: 327 calories

Mid-Afternoon—Meal 4

6 hard-boiled egg whites: 0 grams of fat, 0 grams of carbs, 22 grams of protein

½ ounce of walnuts: 9 grams of fat, 2 grams of carbs, 2 grams of protein

5 cups mixed vegetables: 0 grams of fat, 25 grams of carbs, 0 grams of protein

1 tablespoon vinaigrette: 4 grams of fat, 1½ grams of carbs, 0 grams of protein

13:28½:24

Fat: 117 calories
Carbs: 114 calories

---

*20 calories per cup of mixed vegetables is a rough estimate.

Protein: 96 calories

Total: 327 calories

Dinner—Meal 5

    1 palm-sized serving of baked salmon: 7 grams of fat, 0 grams of carbs,
      25 grams of protein

    ½ cup yellow squash: 0 grams of fat, 3 grams of carbs, 0 grams of
      protein

    ½ cup zucchini: 0 grams of fat, 3 grams of carbs, 0 grams of protein

    ½ cup wild rice: 0 grams of fat, 14 grams of carbs, 3 grams of protein

    1 teaspoon olive oil: 5 grams of fat, 0 grams of carbs, 0 grams of
      protein

    12:20:28

    Fat: 108 calories

    Carbs: 80 calories

    Protein: 112 calories

    Total: 300 calories

    Daily total: 1,537 calories with Breakfast #1; 1,581 calories with Breakfast #2

A personal favorite is to throw a piece of meat on my knockoff George Foreman grill and cut up a variety of raw vegetables, such as yellow, red, and green bell peppers, tomatoes, cucumbers, avocado, mushrooms, broccoli, et cetera. If I don't have much fat in my meat, I'll add a tablespoon of flaxseed oil or olive oil to my veggies. It's easy and delicious, just how I like it.

You're free to rearrange these menus as you see fit and to swap out ingredients and meals entirely. Use this as a starting point. Make it as easy as possible on yourself.

For the first couple of weeks, plan your meals, make shopping lists, and keep a diary of everything you eat. It's a bit of a hassle because of the planning, but you'll see that it soon becomes second nature, as you get familiar with your favorite foods, portion sizes, and timeline.

Look, you don't need a CPA in crunching calories. Meals don't need to be precise. And in the real world, they rarely are. For myself, I simply ensure that I have about a palm-sized portion of protein, carbs coming mostly from raw vegetables, and a little bit of fat. I say a little bit of fat only because it is a calorie-dense macronutrient, so by volume it doesn't take much. Trust me, you'll get the hang of it in no time.

HOOYA!

Here's the Poop

Imagine it's summertime. You had a great barbecue a few days ago. Everyone had an absolute blast. In fact, you had such a blast you forgot to put away the leftovers. So here you are a few days later, walking by your grill, and next to it you find some hamburger patties that have been rotting in 99-degree heat for days on end. Would you:

A. Chow down.
B. Get rid of them.

Seems like a stupid question, huh? Pretty disgusting, actually. Well, if you haven't had a good bowel movement in a few days, then you might as well have eaten those hamburgers, because that's essentially what's in your body.

All the food you eat sits in your intestines at 98.6 degrees, and unless you're regular, you're carrying several days' worth of partially digested, chewed-up, rotting food, rather than only a day's portion.

If you want to feel, look, and perform your best, you have to be regular.

The best way to do this? Drink plenty of water and, whenever possible, replace processed carbs with natural sources like whole pieces of high-fiber fruit and raw veggies. Processed carbs tend to be low in fiber and turn to a thick, sticky paste in your intestines, which can hinder normal removal of waste.

Up until 2011, the government's nutritional guidelines stipulated that half our calories should come from grain products such as breads, rice, corn, and pasta. On a 2,000-calorie diet, that's 365,000 annual calories' worth of low-value, intestine-clogging paste that slowly accumulates inside your body. Now consider how many years you've been on such a diet.

Do whatever it takes to get yourself into the daily habit of eliminating the waste in your intestines before it has a chance to sit and rot. The movement from regular exercise is extremely helpful to this process. Or sometimes it's just a matter of having a little time to yourself, even in the privacy of your own home, for your body to get in the mood.

The gradual buildup of waste and toxins in the intestines can cause bloating, bad skin, and eventually irritable bowel syndrome, among other things. There are myriad health reasons to get regular. Your energy will increase, nutrients will absorb properly, appetite will be regulated, your weight and waistline will immediately decrease, and, with a good strength program like mine, fat will start coming off your body much more easily.

Your awareness of what you eat and how you eat will quickly become unconscious. But you must train yourself to get to this point.

Common Female Deficiencies

As you read labels and plan your meals, keep in mind that many women don't consume enough of certain micronutrients. Be mindful of the following common areas of deficiency:

CALCIUM

Eighty percent of people suffering from osteoporosis are female. Low levels of calcium often do not become apparent until later in life, when the slow loss of bone mass causes a decrease in quality of life due to a brittle and injury-prone skeletal system. One of the benefits of strength training is the increase in bone density, but the full effect of this can't be realized without adequate calcium absorption.

VITAMIN D3

This nutrient plays a vital role in the absorption of calcium. It also plays an important role in the maintenance of the nervous and immune systems. Certain types of cancers, such as breast, ovarian, colon, and bladder, have been associated with vitamin D3 deficiencies.

Vitamin D3 deficiencies are especially common in those climates where sunlight is scarce. D3 is created in your skin mainly during exposure to sunlight. Fair-skinned people are much more efficient at producing D3 from sunlight than are those with dark skin. Vitamin D3 is of such importance that it actually caused people in northern climates to evolve to have lighter skin.

As a general rule, it's healthy to expose at least a quarter of your unprotected skin to direct sunlight for five to fifteen minutes, three to four times per week. Those with lighter skin need less exposure, while those with darker skin need more.

ACIDIC DIETS

The body needs to maintain slightly alkaline blood for optimal health. When our diets cause us to become slightly acidic instead, the body uses calcium and other minerals to neutralize the acids, and these minerals can come from both our diets and our bones. Most people's pH levels on Western diets are acidic, mainly because they eat too much meat and dairy and too few vegetables. This, too, can be corrected by getting most of your carbs from a variety of vegetables and fruits and by taking a greens supplement, such as Green Vibrance, that is alkalinizing due to the vegetation from which it's made.

IRON

Due to menstrual cycles, many women are iron deficient. This can lead to chronic feelings of fatigue and poor training performance. Eating iron-rich foods such as liver and red meats, preparing foods using cast-iron cookware, and taking an iron supplement help to correct this deficiency. If you take a greens supplement that contains iron, I suggest taking two servings a day the week of your cycle.

OMEGA-3 TO OMEGA-6 RATIO

In his book *Anticancer: A New Way of Life*, David Servan-Schreiber, MD, PhD, points out that, between 1976 and 2000, Americans lowered fat consumption by 11 percent and calorie intake by 4 percent, yet obesity went up 31 percent in this same period.

In addition to inactivity and processed carbs, a likely cause is the omega-3 to omega-6 ratio, which is severely out of balance in Western diets. What should be a 1:1 omega-3 to omega-6 ratio is anywhere from 1:15 to 1:30 in most.

This imbalance is due to the large consumption of vegetable oils and products from livestock that are fed grains, corn, and soy instead of grass. The food that makes our livestock fat is also making us fat, because of the omega imbalances they cause. These fatty acids cannot be produced in the body and must come from food sources.

The solution is to eat plenty of fish and products derived from livestock that is grass fed (1:1 ratio) and to avoid as much as possible the "heart healthy" vegetable oil contained in almost all processed foods. Flaxseed oil, olive oil, coconut oil, and fish oil are great sources of dietary fat, and they also help to correct this imbalance.

9

The Top Ten Ways to Gain as Much Fat as Possible!*

10. Don't Break Fast

Study after study has shown that women who don't eat breakfast are more overweight than those who do. After about eight hours of fasting, it's important *not* to kick-start your metabolism by eating. This way you can lose muscle while gaining fat. And at the same time you can ensure that cravings instead of smart choices determine your diet.

Definitely avoid eating a little piece of fresh, hydrating fruit immediately after you wake up. The sugar from the fruit will likely spur your appetite within twenty to thirty minutes and make it more difficult to skip the most crucial meal of the day.

9. Starve Yourself

Avoid eating small regular meals that will keep you energized and satisfied. Rather than eating a small meal about every three hours, stick with just a couple of big ones that create a sugar rush and crash after a strong insulin reaction. Starving yourself is a great way to ensure your calorie-burning muscles aren't provided a steady flow of needed nutrients, so they can wither and make room for new fat.

---

*Obviously, please do the exact opposite of these ten steps! Then you're good to go!

8. Eat High-Glycemic Carbs

More than anything else, consuming massive amounts of processed carbs with high glycemic indices has led to Western civilization's obesity problem. Everything from whole-wheat bread, yogurts, sports bars, fruit juices, cereals, and sodas contain large amounts of high-glycemic carbs.

To gain fat, eat only carbs with glycemic indices well above 55. And, if at all possible, eat these processed carbs by themselves. This will maximize the blood-sugar spike and crash. Protein and especially fat slow the absorption of sugars, which is *not* what you need to get *huge*.

7. Avoid Raw Vegetables and High-Fiber Fruits

These are your number one enemy because of their high nutritional value, high volume-to-calorie ratio, and slow rate of absorption. Most vegetables and fruits contain things like vitamins, minerals, fiber, and water. What they do not contain is a lot of calories. Consider that two cups of yellow squash and zucchini are only 40 calories. Just 400 calories from most raw vegetables will require that you eat at least 20 cups' worth! It's kind of hard to gain weight this way.

By replacing your current raw vegetables and high-fiber fruits with processed carbs, you will get more empty calories, which are sure to keep you hungry and dissatisfied due to insulin surges and micronutrient deficiencies.

6. Avoid Water

Instead, drink fruit juices and sodas. Most juices have about 115 calories of high-glycemic sugar in each cup. A can of soda has about 140 calories. You can really rack up the empty calories with these. Best of all, your blood-sugar levels will spike and crash all day. Diet sodas are pretty good, too, since artificial sweeteners are linked to metabolic disorders and increased cravings for sweets.

Monitor your urine and make sure it comes out in all sorts of funky colors! If it's clear, that means you've accidentally hydrated yourself with water.

5. Eat Fast and Furious

It takes your body about twenty minutes to realize how full it is, so it's important to get as much food into your mouth as fast as you can. Eating only one or two meals a day makes this much easier, since you'll be starving by the time you finally eat.

4. Stay Away from Foods That Are Whole

The mixing of ingredients needs to occur in factories and not in your kitchen. When you shop, purchase only processed foods that contain tons of ingredients. Make sure you can *not* pronounce all of them. These foods have the most calories, highest glycemic indices, and lowest nutritional value. Definitely avoid shopping the perimeter of your grocery store, where single-ingredient items might distract you—such as fruits, veggies, red meats, poultry, fish, eggs, nuts, and seeds.

3. Maintain a Caloric Excess

Consume 500 to 750 calories more than you expend each day. Most women looking to gain significant amounts of fat will do well on 3,000 calories a day, twice that of someone looking to lose fat. An efficient way to pack on the pounds is to eat fried or battered food.

And whatever you do, *don't* go to YouAreYourOwnGym.com and use the resting metabolism calculator under the "Nutrition" link, which tells you your caloric needs based on your specific goals (losing fat, toning, or filling out your body). Just eat, eat, eat up!

2. Diet 'til You Drop

If you do get duped into a fat-loss diet, I strongly recommend *never* taking a break from it. Normally, with other people, I recommend upping the calories a bit for seven days of every month, to maintain a caloric balance. This prevents overtraining, burnout, and a loss of strength. It can also keep your morale high and maintain your sanity. But, please, forget about little things like sanity, and keep on nonstop dieting as long as you possibly can, until you finally fall off the wagon for good.

1. Don't Build Muscle

Avoid physical activity! If you must exercise, stick to low-intensity aerobic activity, which won't build muscle, will possibly cause muscle wasting, and won't have a lasting metabolic effect.

The Final Step: Independence

You have a choice: Take care of yourself, or put the effort off until it's too late. And it is right now, at this moment, not later, no matter what else is happening in your life, that you must make this decision.

Most people in this world choose to lose. They drag themselves through a second-rate life, overweight and under-energetic. They let time take its toll. Their waistline increases and their height decreases as they get older, and their backs hurt and hunch. Eventually their mobility becomes limited. And often they meet their maker well before they should.

Then there are the others, the minority, *us*, who decide to really, truly do something about our health. We exercise, and we watch what we eat—not obsessively, only just enough. We have an understanding of nutritional basics and work out twenty to thirty minutes a day, three times a week—less than one percent of our time—because that is all we will ever need. We meet life's obstacles with physical, mental, and spiritual strength. We care about how we look, and we look good.

We thrive on the energy exercise gives us every day, how it washes away so many of the bad things in life—depression, anxiety, nervousness, tension, boredom, impatience. . . . It lets us think easily and clearly. We know how much worse our lives would be if we did not exercise, so we simply don't let that happen.

Having an athletic body is one of the greatest secrets to a happier life.

And now, finally, you can achieve that with little sacrifice to your time. Your new athleticism blends into the life you already have and lets you enjoy it all the more.

But there is no room for tourists here. If you want to lose weight and look great, you have to do more than one four-week program. You have to make these exercises and nutritional guidance part of your life. You must go all the way with this book, or you'll end up going none of the way.

Ninety-nine percent of the truly fit women I know accomplish their fitness on their own. Others take classes, hire trainers, or find workout partners, because they want to be motivated or held accountable. Sure, it can be nice having a teacher or trainer offer reassurance, pat you on the back, or even scold you when you need it. But ultimately no one can hold you accountable but you.

You need to build full independence into your regimen to be successful over the long term. Only *you* know what you need and when you need it. Only *you* feel your muscles, lungs, bones, and ligaments. In the end, only you can get you into shape. And now that's *all* you need—*you*—to work out effectively when you're by yourself, whenever you want, wherever you want, for the rest of your life.

Women today are in charge of so many things—from the largest global corporations to military commands to households (and, no, that's not in descending order of importance). But too many do not exercise control over their selves.

Just before the turn of the twentieth century, Susan B. Anthony declared, "The bicycle has done more to emancipate women than anything else in the world." She sang the praises of an athletic device that gave women newfound freedom and self-reliance. Now, after the turn of the twenty-first century, we're finally taking the next step. Now a woman needs nothing but herself to become leaner and stronger than ever before. This is real freedom. Real self-reliance. Final independence.

Independence in your fitness is the true theme to this book. It is the number one secret to lifelong good looks and health.

You're there for everyone else, but you must first be there for yourself. No one in this world can instill true motivation in you except you. Ultimate fitness is not achieved by depending on a community. There's only one thing you can depend on . . . one thing you are never without: You.

You are your own driving force.

You are your own gym.

Acknowledgments

I'd like to thank my loving girlfriend, Samantha, for her tremendous support. Taking her from her first Let Me In to her first Pull-up has been a rewarding experience. Thank you, baby.

I'd also like to thank Jeannie, our model, for the incredible energy and time she devoted to the photo shoots. As a wife, professional mother, and now an athelete and a friend, she is an inspiration.

Last but not least, both authors would like to thank the two people who made this book a reality. Our editor, Marnie Cochran, took all our long, hard work and honed it into a singular vision. We couldn't have a better editor. And we can't thank our agent, Steve Ross, enough, for his continued guidance and partnership.

About the Authors

MARK LAUREN is a military physical training specialist for the Special Operations community, a sought-after personal trainer to civilian men and women of all fitness levels, a triathlete, a champion Thai boxer, and the author of the internationally popular body-weight bible *You Are Your Own Gym*. He lives in Tampa, Florida.

www.YouAreYourOwnGym.com

JOSHUA CLARK is the author of *Heart Like Water: Surviving Katrina and Life in Its Disaster Zone*, a finalist for the National Book Critics Circle Award. The founder of Light of New Orleans Publishing, he has edited such books as *French Quarter Fiction*; *Southern Fried Divorce, Louisiana: In Words*; and *How You Can Kill Al Qaeda (in 3 Easy Steps)*. He is also a certified personal trainer, who has not set foot in a gym since Hurricane Katrina closed his fitness center.

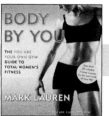

GOALS

_____

_____

_____

_____

_____

_____

_____

_____

_____

_____

_____

_____

_____

_____

_____

_____

EXCUSES

_____

_____

_____

_____

_____

_____

_____

_____

_____

_____

_____

_____

_____

_____

_____

_____

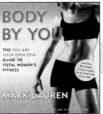

GOALS

EXCUSES

_____

_____

_____

_____

_____

_____

_____

_____

_____

_____

_____

_____

_____

_____

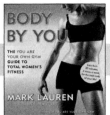

_____   _____

_____   _____

_____   _____

_____   _____

_____   _____

_____   _____

_____   _____

_____   _____

_____   _____

_____   _____

_____   _____

_____   _____

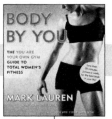

GOALS

EXCUSES

_____
_____
_____
_____
_____
_____
_____
_____
_____
_____
_____
_____
_____
_____
_____
_____

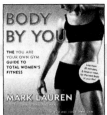

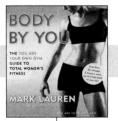

_____

_____

_____

_____

_____

_____

_____

_____

_____

_____

_____

_____

_____

_____

_____

_____

GOALS

EXCUSES

GOALS

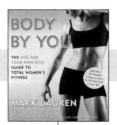

EXCUSES

_____

_____

_____

_____

_____

_____

_____

_____

_____

_____

_____

_____

_____

_____

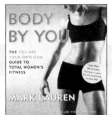

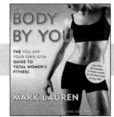

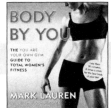

THIS IS ME BEFORE I STARTED *BODY BY YOU*

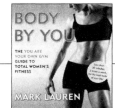

THIS IS ME AFTER TWO MONTHS OF *BODY BY YOU* WORKOUTS